The Best of Srilankan Food Recipes

Healthy Cooking with Coconut and Spices

SHRINIKA PERERA

Copyright © 2014 by Shrinika Perera

All rights reserved. No part of this book may be reproduced or transmitted in any form or by any means, electronic or mechanical, including photocopying, recording, or by any information storage and retrieval system, without permission in writing from the copyright owner.

Print information available on the last page.

Rev. date: 04/17/2015

www.bestofsrilankanfood.com

Table of Contents

DEDICATION 1

THE BEST OF SRI LANKAN FOOD 2

Breakfasts 13

    MILK RICE 14

    MUNG KIRIBATH- (MILK RICE WITH GREEN GRAM) 15

    POLL MALLUN (SWEET COCONUT AND HONEY MIX) 16

    IMBUL KIRIBATH 17

    PITTU 18

    ROTI 21

    ONION AND GREEN CHILLI ROTTI 22

    HOPPERS- (AAPPER) 24

    STRING HOPPERS 26

    LUNUMIRIS 28

    CHICKEN CURRY 31

    KIRI HODI 33

    POTATO CURRY 35

    FISH AMBUL THIAL 37

    COCONUT SAMBAL 38

    TEMPERED DHAL CURRY 41

    SEENI SAMBOL 43

Rice 46

    YELLOW RICE PILAU WITH CHICKEN 47

- FRIED RICE 49
- LUMP RICE 51

Curries and Salads 53
- EGG SALAD 54
- CUTLETS 56
- FRIED POTATOES 58
- BEANS CURRY 60
- EGGPLANT MODJU/ WAMBATU MODJU 62
- CASHEW CURRY 64
- SINHALA ACHCHARU-PICKLE 66
- PINEAPPLE CURRY 68
- POLLOS CURRY 70
- FRIED DHAMBALA CURRY 73
- BRINJAL PAHIE 75
- PUMPKIN WITH ROASTED COCONUT CURRY 78

Seafood and Fish 81
- DEVILLED PRAWNS 82
- FRIED FISH 85
- PRAWNS CURRY 87
- CRAB CURRY 90
- FISH CURRY - (THORA MALU FISH CURRY) 93
- FRIED DRIED FISH 95

Dinner Ideas 97
- TEMPERED MANIOC OR CASSAVA WITH FISH CURRY 98
- KOTTU ROTI 101

Desserts..104
    WATALAPPUM..105
    CHOCOLATE MARIE BISCUIT PUDDING.......................107

DEDICATION

This book is dedicated to my beloved parents, my husband, and daughter for their co-operation in realizing my dream.

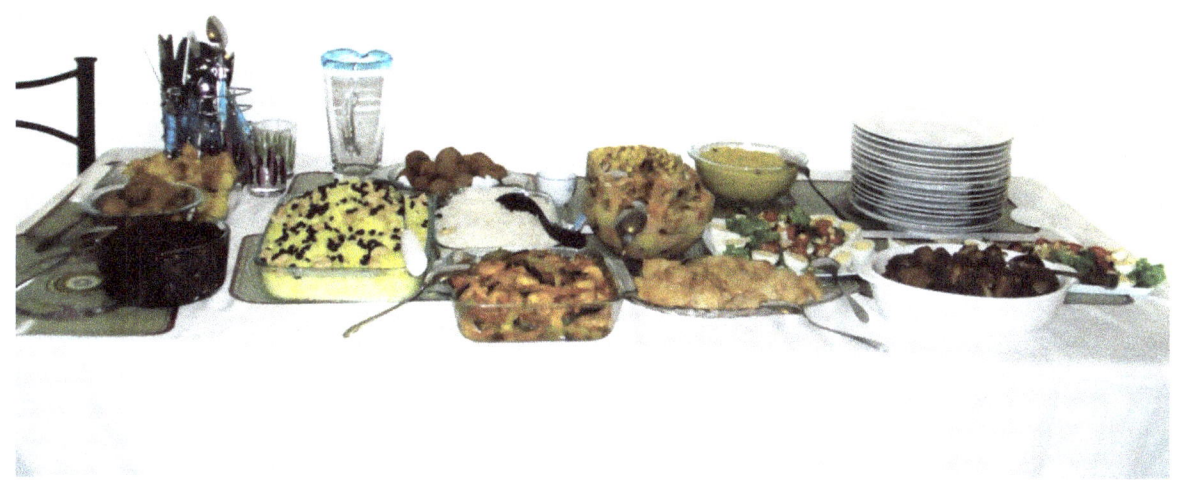

THE BEST OF SRI LANKAN FOOD

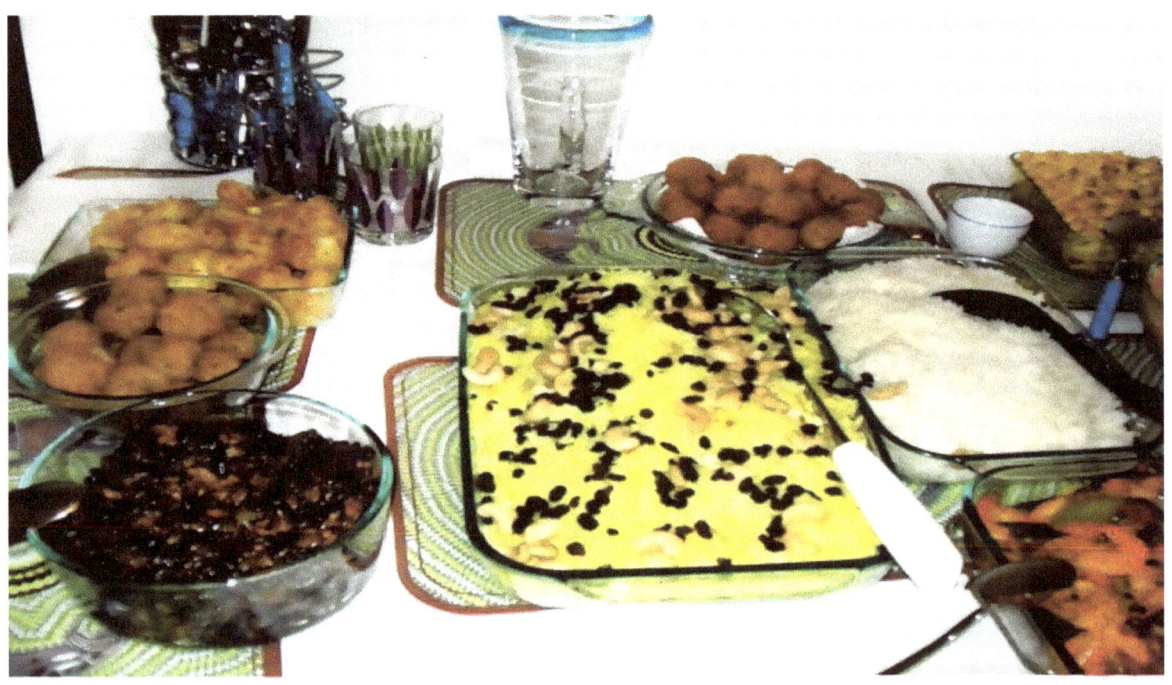

Sri Lanka is one of the most beautiful countries in the world, and because of its beauty, it is called the Pearl of the Indian Ocean or Paradise. Often called one of the best tourist attractions in the world, Sri Lanka has pristine beaches, a tropical climate, natural beauty, ancient history, and best of all, delicious cuisine.

I lived on this beautiful island for over 35 years before migrating to Australia. While I'm a certified accountant, I am more excited when I use my spare time to cook. I had a passion for cooking since my childhood. During those years, I helped my mother, as well as my grandmother, prepare traditional Sri Lankan dishes. I can remember the mouth-watering food my grandmother prepared and served us on many visits to her home during long school holidays. Over time, I learned little-known secrets about traditional Sri Lankan cooking from my mother, my grandmother, as well as from my family and friends.

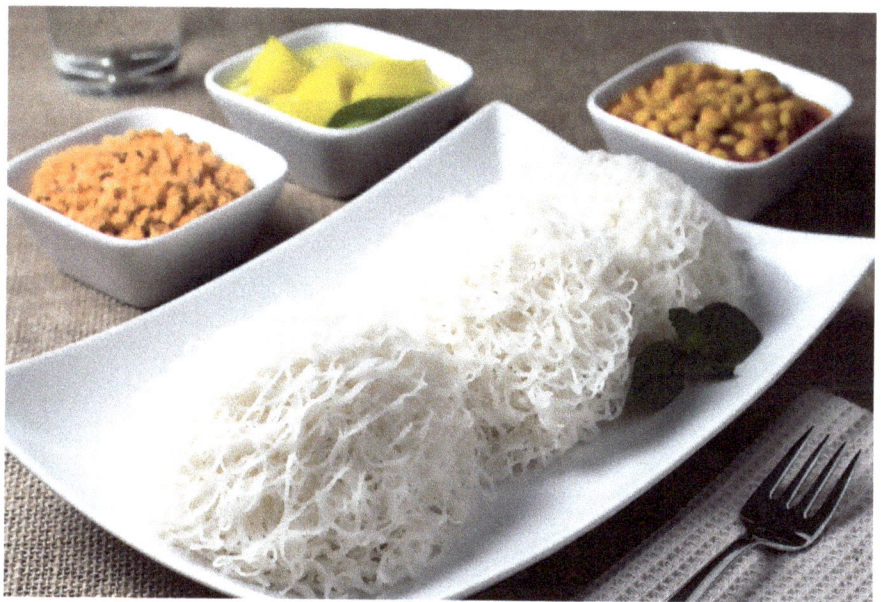

The goal of "The Best of Sri Lankan Food Recipes" is to introduce the little-known secrets about Sri Lankan cuisine to a wider audience. The recipes I have carefully selected will enlighten and entertain both the Western and Asians taste buds. These recipes use healthy ingredients such as coconut oil, coconut milk, coconut flakes, and spices to add authentic Sri Lankan flavors.

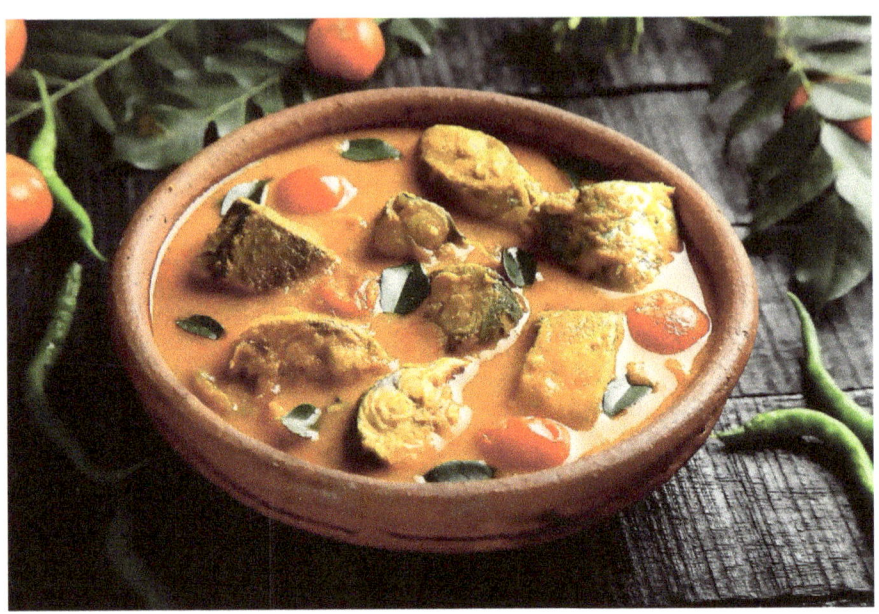

Coconut oil is used extensively in tropical countries, especially in India, Sri Lanka, Thailand, and the Philippines, as they enjoy the yearlong production of the oil. Coconut oil is one of the foods classified as a "superfood." This designation is due to its unique combination of fatty acids that have profound positive effects on health. At one time, the oil was also popular in western countries, like the United States and Canada.

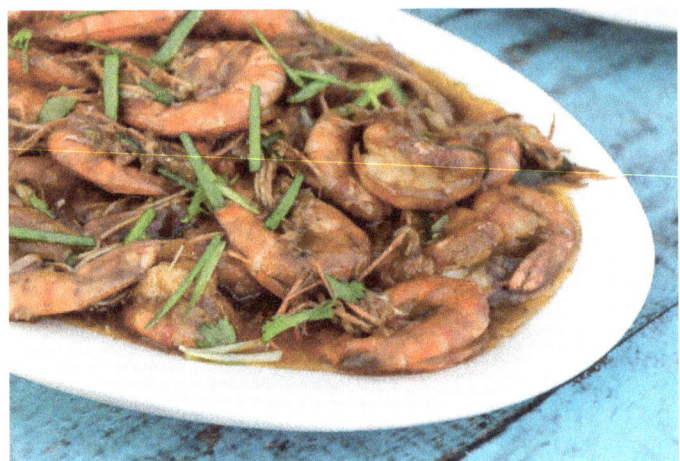

According to current research, coconut oil contains fewer calories than other oils, and its fat content is easily converted into energy. In addition, it does not lead to an accumulation of fat in the heart and arteries. Coconut oil also helps boost energy and endurance and can enhance the performance of athletes.

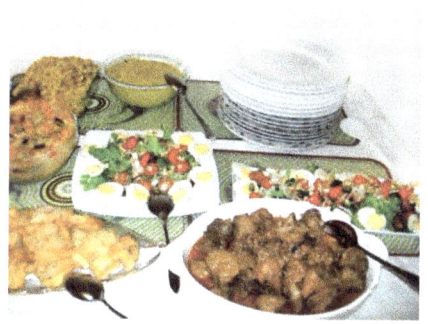 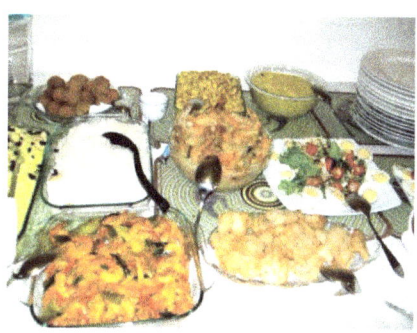

Coconut oil is beneficial for the heart. It contains about 50% lauric acid, which helps prevent various heart problems, like high cholesterol levels and high blood pressure. The saturated fats present in coconut oil are not harmful, unlike the ones you find in vegetable oils. Coconut oil is very useful for weight loss. It contains short and medium-chain fatty acids that aid in removing excess weight. This oil is also easy to digest, and it helps in supporting the healthy function of the thyroid and endocrine system. Further, it increases the body's metabolic rate by removing stress on the pancreas, thereby burning more energy and helping obese and overweight people lose weight. People who use coconut oil every day as their primary cooking oil are normally not fat, obese, or overweight.

As mentioned before, this book is filled with different recipes with coconut oil, coconut milk, coconut flakes, and spices authentic to build Sri Lankan flavors. Coconut oils, coconut flakes, dried coconut milk powder, and Sri Lankan spices are available in Asian grocery stores. Coconut milk cans/tins, coconut water, and spices are available in any supermarket.

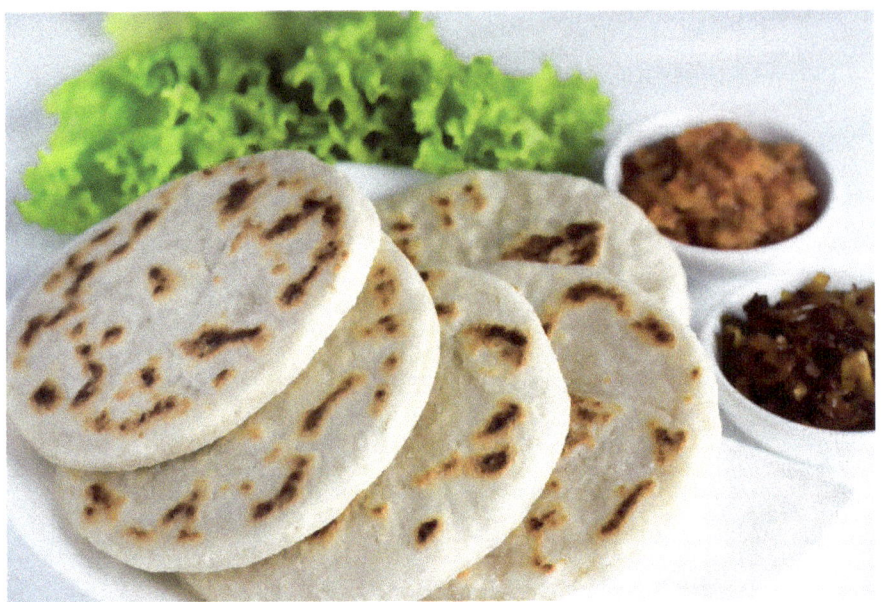

This book is perfect for:

- Someone looking for the correct method of traditional Sri Lankan cooking.
- Great new ideas for delicious home-made meals;
- Planning your menus and accompaniments, or
- A novice cook

Every recipe has been tried and tested numerous times with my family and friends. As a result, this book will give you consistent, delicious results for creating mouth-watering meals. Some of these recipes will be everyday family recipes, and others will come in handy planning for a family feast or small dinner party. Some of the recipes are my own creations. These recipes include serving ideas, so it's simple to plan your menus with serving dishes. This book has everything you need to make sure you're serving the best for your family and friends.

Some of Sri Lankans' favorite foods are Hoppers, String Hoppers, Lump Rice, Koththu Roti, and Fried rice and their accompanying curries. These foods are authentic to Sri Lankans, which is likely why they're now popular worldwide and enjoyed in Australia, the USA, and the UK. Anyone who has visited Sri Lanka or has tried these foods before will recognize the mouth-watering flavors and would love to try these recipes for their own.

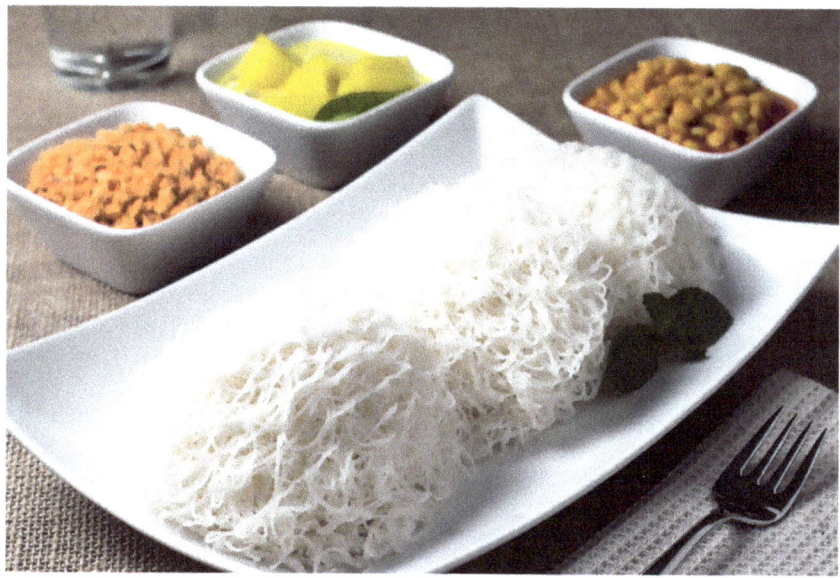

This book offers a gold mine of little-known secrets about Sri Lankan cooking that will give you the confidence you need. You now have the correct recipes, the correct ingredients, and step-by-step instructions to lead you to the ideal dishes.

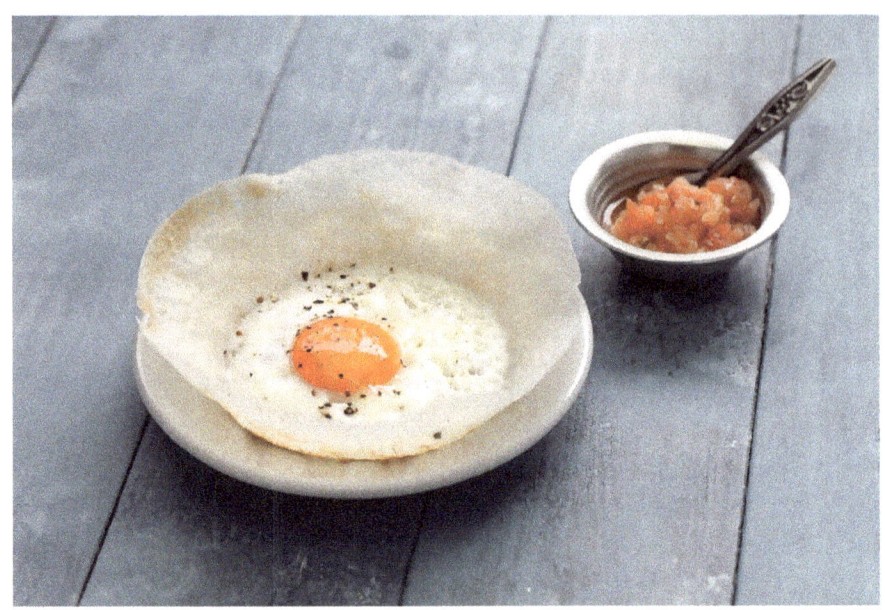

Another purpose of this book is to help others learn and experience Sri Lankan flavors without any difficulty. Even if someone feels cooking Sri Lankan food is difficult, they will begin to see cooking these dishes isn't as hard as they thought.

Sri Lankan food is similar to Indian food, but the big difference is that Sri Lankans prefer coconut milk over yogurt for making sauces and curries.

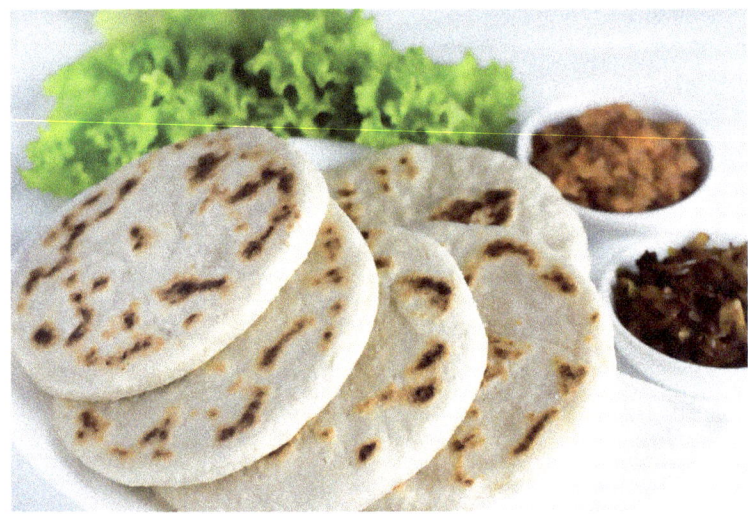

These sensational recipes are presented in a simple format so that even a novice in the kitchen will easily understand and try their hand in cooking delicious meals.

Although individual tastes may vary, color, fragrance, and presentation are important. My secrets of tasty cooking include knowing the correct measurements and recipes, proper planning, fresh ingredients, and the right utensils.

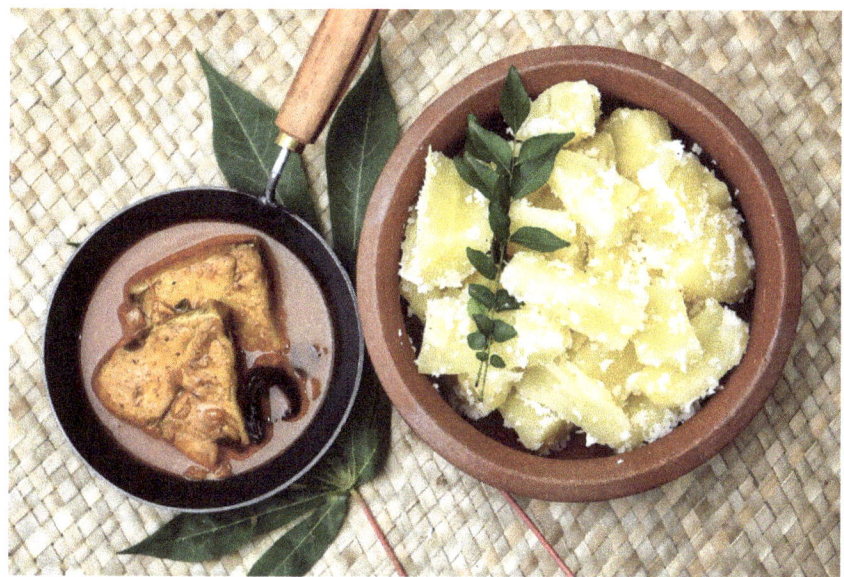

Even for a novice, my advice is not to stress when it comes to making Sri Lankan food. Even if you don't have all the ingredients like Rampe, Goraka (Gamboge), Curry leaves, or Maldive fish, don't stress. Simply try the recipe without them.

This book will give you the confidence to cook Sri Lankan recipes the correct way.

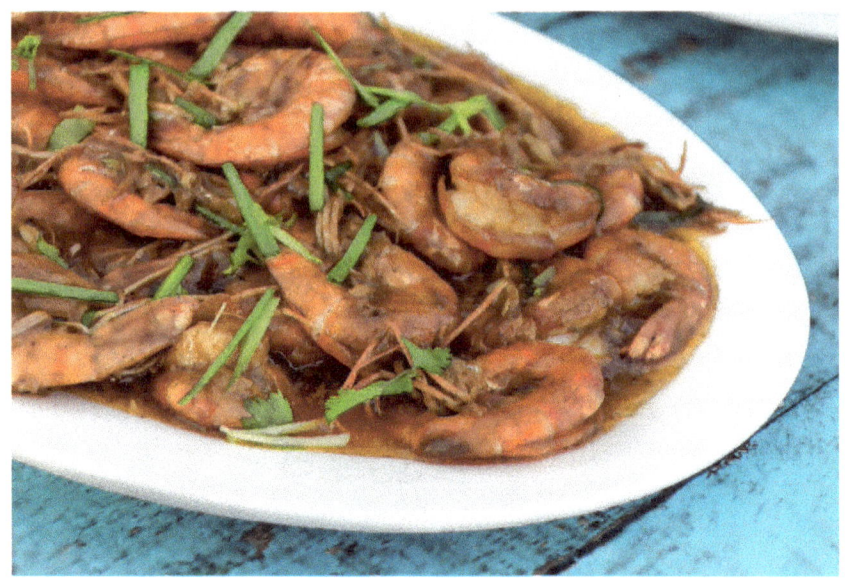

I hope you enjoy learning the little-known secrets about Sri Lankan cooking, I know you will achieve your desired flavors, and I know you can overcome your fears of cooking these special dishes.

I have included colored photos in most of the recipes to help you understand what these foods might look like, allowing you to focus on the cooking and taste. If I make you hungry as you read, I have accomplished my true goal: to share my joy of cooking.

Enjoy your 'travels' to Sri Lanka!

WEIGHTS AND MEASURES

Dry ingredients		Liquids	
METRIC	IMPERIAL	METRIC	IMPERIAL
15g	1/2oz	30ml	1 fl.oz
30g	1oz	60ml	2fl.oz (1/4 cup)
60g	2oz	100ml	3fl.oz
90g	3oz	125ml (1/2 cup)	4fl.oz (1/2 cup)
125g	4oz (1/4 lb)	150ml	5fl.oz (1/4 pt)
155g	5oz	185ml (3/4 cup)	6fl.oz (3/4 cup)
185g	6oz	250ml (1 cup)	8fl.oz (1 cup)
220g	7oz	300ml (1 ¼ cups)	10fl.oz (1/2 pt)
250g	8oz (1/2 lb)	360ml (1 ½ cups)	12fl.oz (1 ½ cups)
280g	9oz	420ml (1 ¾ cups)	14fl.oz (1 ¾ cups)
315g	10oz	500ml (2 cups)	16fl.oz (2 cups)
345g	11oz	625ml (2 ½ cups)	20fl.oz (1 pt)
375g	12oz (3/4 lb)	1000ml/ 1L (4 cups)	
410g	13oz	ml- millilitres	
440g	14oz	L- Litre	
470g	15oz	fl.oz-fluid ounce	
500g (0.5kg)	16oz (1 lb)		
750g (.75kg)	24oz (1 ½ lbs)		
1000g (1 kg)	32oz (2 lbs)		
g- grams			
kg- kilograms			
oz- ounces			
lbs- pounds			

OVEN TEMPERATURES

	Celsius	Fahrenheit	Gas Mark
Very slow	120	250	½
Slow	140-150	275-300	1-2
Moderately slow	160	325	3
Moderate	180	350	4
Moderately hot	190	375	5
Hot	200	400	6
	220	425	7
	230	450	8
Very Hot	250-260	475-500	9

Some of the commonly used spices with Sri Lankan words are here for your guidance

Capsicums-Malu Miris

Cardamoms- Karadhamungu/Enasal

Chilli-Miris

Cloves-Karabu Nati

Coconut flakesCoconut Milk- Pol KiriCoconut Oil- Pol Thell

Coriander-Kothamalli

Cumin-Suduru

Curry Leaves-Karapincha

Dried coconut milk powder

Fennel Seeds-Maduru

Fenugreek-Uluhaal

Gamboge-Goraka

Jaggery-Hakuru

Lemongrass-Sera

Maldive Fish-Umbalakade

Mustard Seeds-Aba

Pandanus-Rampe

Tamarind-Siyambala

Turmeric Powder-Kaha

BREAKFASTS

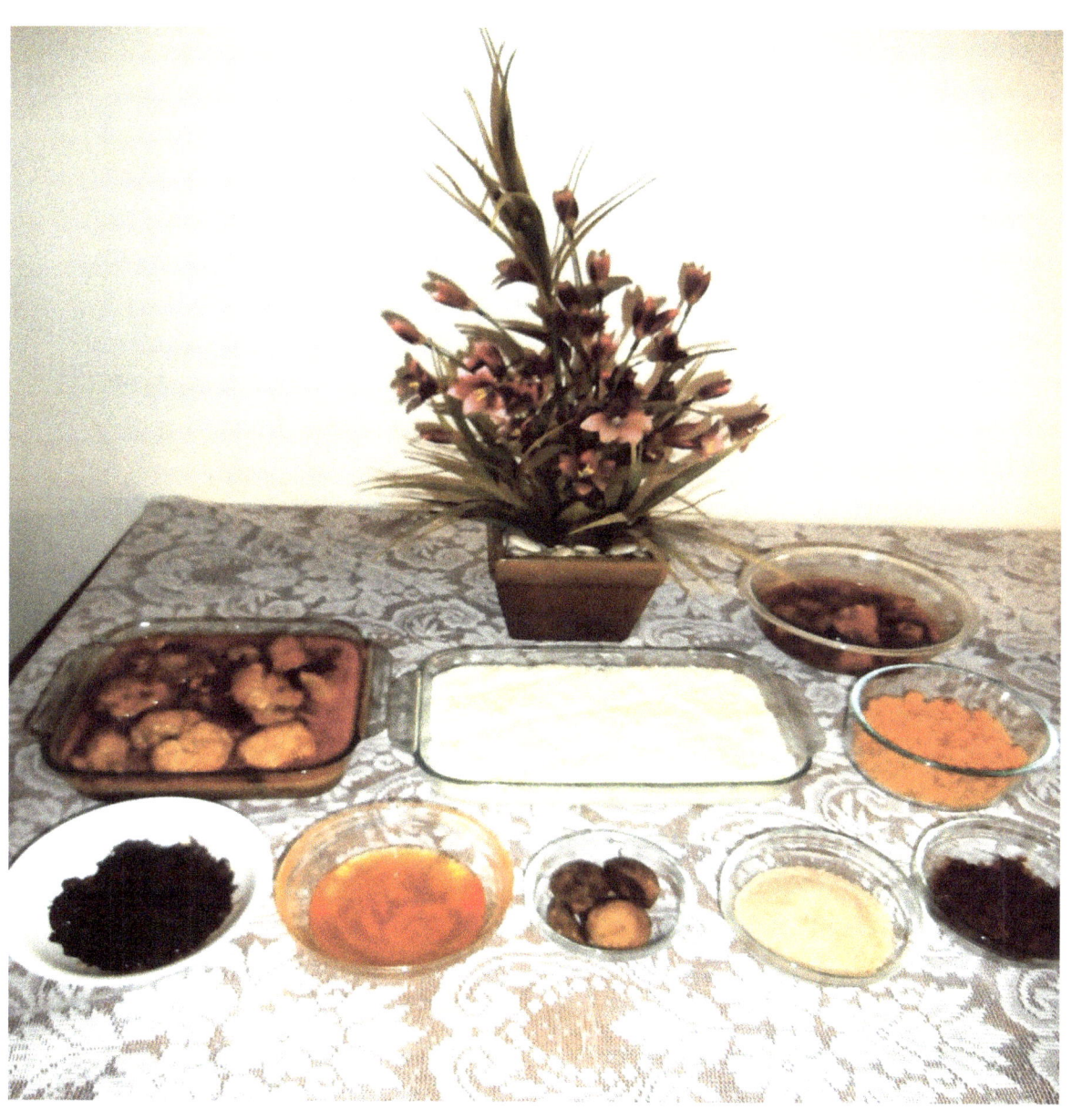

MILK RICE

Ingredients:

- 250g Red or White Kakulu / any Raw Rice
- 2 Cups Thick coconut milk or 1 Tin thick coconut cream (You can use 2 tbsp. Dried coconut milk powder diluted in 1 cup water to make 1 cup thick coconut milk. Dried Coconut Milk is available in Asian grocery shops.)
- Salt to taste
- Water to cook the rice

Method:

Wash the rice. Add sufficient water to cook the rice. When the rice is half cooked, add the tin of coconut cream or the thick coconut milk and salt. Cover and leave on a moderate fire to cook slowly. Mix well all the time until it forms a thick consistency. Spread the rice on to a platter and smooth top with the back of a spoon or banana leaf. When warm, cut into large diamond-shaped or square pieces.

Serving Ideas:

Meat/ Fish or Chicken curries, Lunumiris, Seeni Sambol, Jaggary, Treacle, Bananas, and Katta Sambol.

MUNG KIRIBATH- (MILK RICE WITH GREEN GRAM)

Use the same Milk Rice recipe. Soak about 100 grams of Green Gram for about 2-3 hours. Add the green gram to raw rice, add water, and cook until rice is boiled. Then add the coconut cream or coconut milk and simmer. Spread the rice on to a platter and smooth top with the back of a spoon or banana leaf. When warm, cut into large diamond-shaped or square pieces.

Serving Suggestions:

Lunumiris, Seeni Sambol, Juggary, Treacle, Meat/ Fish or Chicken curries, Bananas, Katta Sambol.

POLL MALLUN (SWEET COCONUT AND HONEY MIX)

Ingredients:

- 200g Scraped Coconut
- 1 ½ Cups Treacle
- 4 Cardamoms- grounded
- 4 Cloves- grounded
- Salt to taste
- Lemon zest

Method:

Add treacle, coconut, grounded cardamoms, and cloves. Cook on slow heat until the coconut is cooked. Add the salt and lemon zest and combine. Use this mixture for the Imbul Kiribath filling.

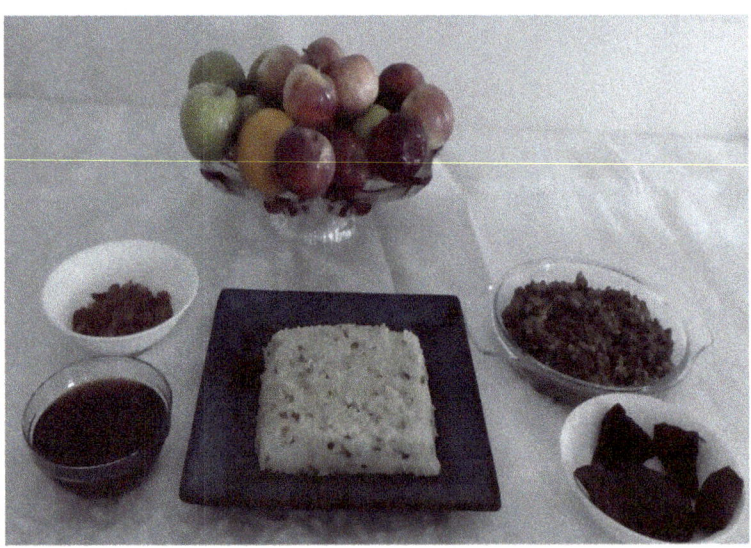

IMBUL KIRIBATH

Place a big lump of milk rice in the middle of a cooking foil or banana leaf and spread in a circular motion. Add poll mallun mixture in the middle. (Recipe is given.) Using the sides of the cooking foil or the banana leaf, fold and twist the mixture into a big roll making the poll mallun settle in the middle. It is very delicious and great for special occasions.

PITTU

Ingredients:

- 225g Roasted Rice Flour (Red or white)
- 225g Scrapped Coconut (Frozen or grated)
- 1tsp Salt to taste
- Water to mix

Method:

Sift the flour. Add the grated coconut and salt to the flour and mix using the tips of the fingers. Sprinkle some water and mix until the mixture resembles small balls or bread crumbs. Mixture should not be sticky in your hands. Fill the mixture in a Pittu Mould. If you like, you can add coconut in between pittu mixture to add flavor before steaming. Steam for about 20 minutes. Take off from steam and push out pittu with a stick onto a plate while hot. Cut into pieces and serve.

Serving Ideas:

Serve with thick coconut milk, Potato Curry, Sugar, Jaggery, Kiri Hodi, Katta Sambal, Lunumiris, Coconut Sambol, and Meat, Fish, Chicken, or vegetable curry.

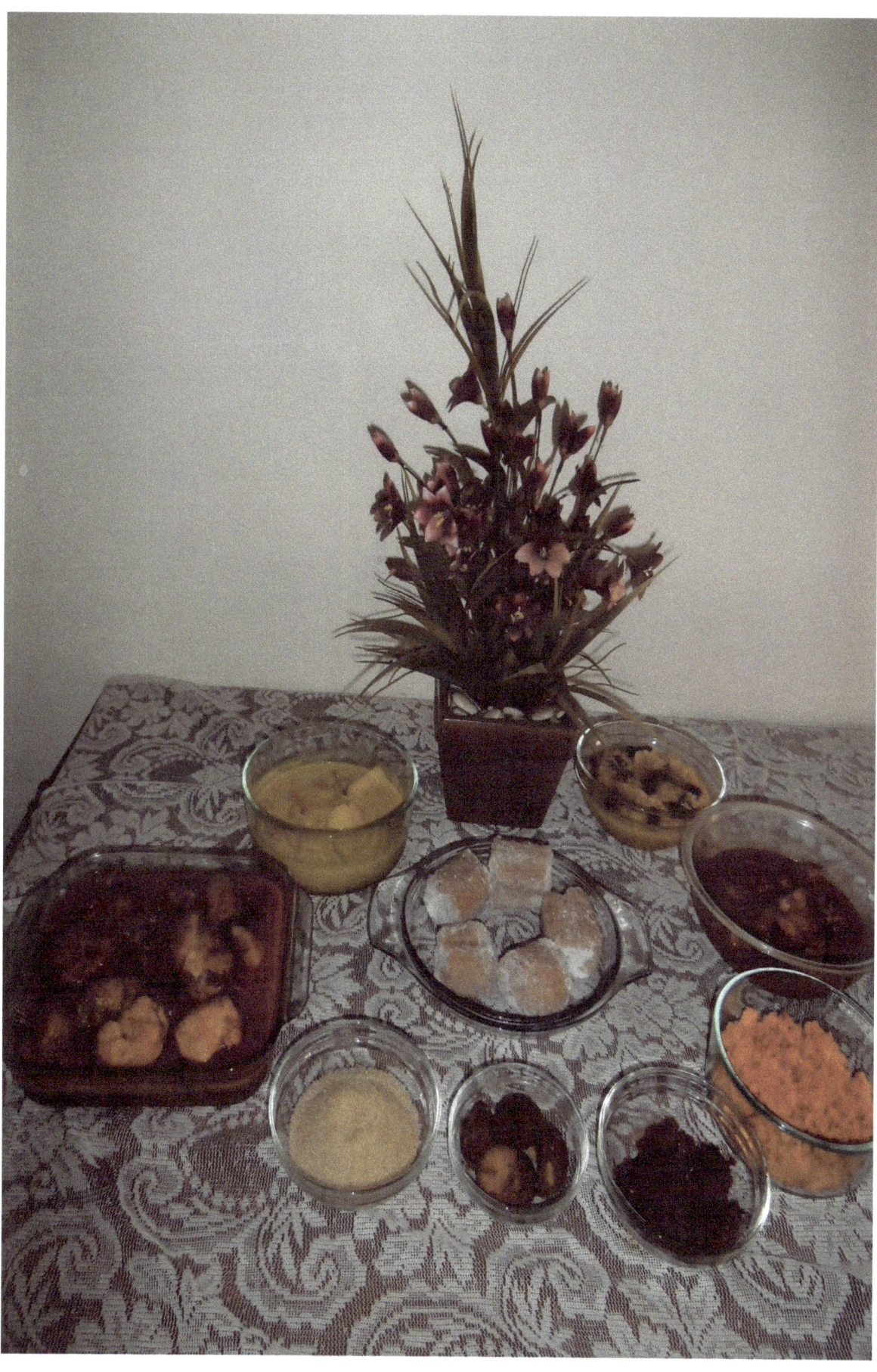

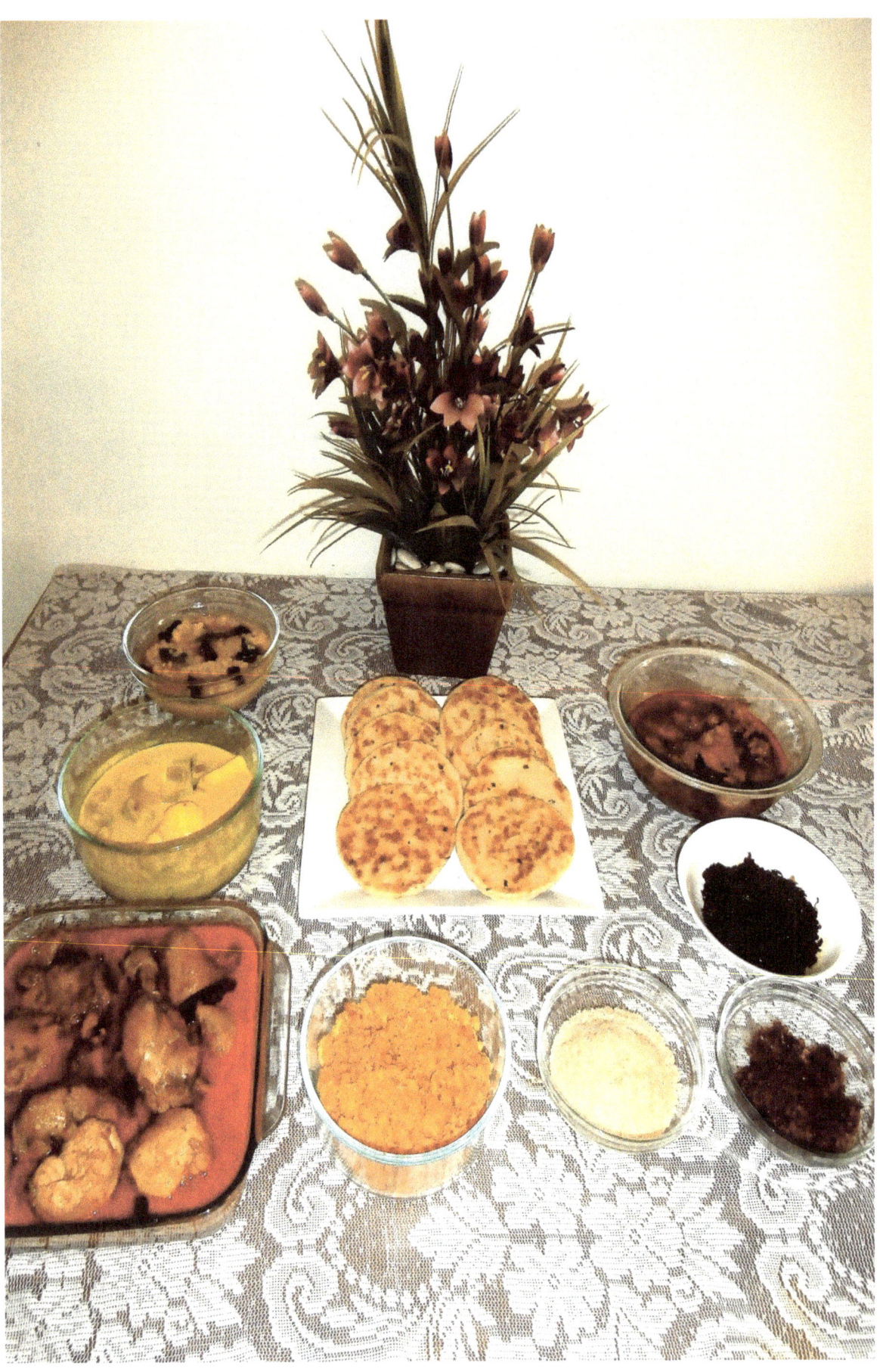

ROTI

Ingredients:

- 250g Plain Flour.
- 250g Scrapped Coconut
- Salt
- Cold Water to mix

Method:

Sift the flour and add the scraped coconut and salt. Mix together and make a soft dough. Knead until dough forms into a ball that will not stick to your hands. Divide the dough into small balls. Flatten each ball on a Banana leaf or on a benchtop to make thin rounds. Cook in a hot griddle or a frying pan. If you like to add more flavor, you can cook the roti on top of a banana leaf. Roast both sides until they turn to golden brown color.

Serve: With Sugar, Lunumiris, Katta Sambol, Fish Ambul Thiyal, Chicken curry, Fish Curry, or Vegetable curry.

Instead of plain flour, you can use lightly roasted red or white rice flour, wholemeal flour, or kurakkan flour to make it healthy.

ONION AND GREEN CHILLI ROTTI

Add a little bit of chopped red onions, green chilies, and a sprig of chopped curry leaves to the basic roti mixture to make it tastier. It could be served with Chicken or fish curry or lunumiris.

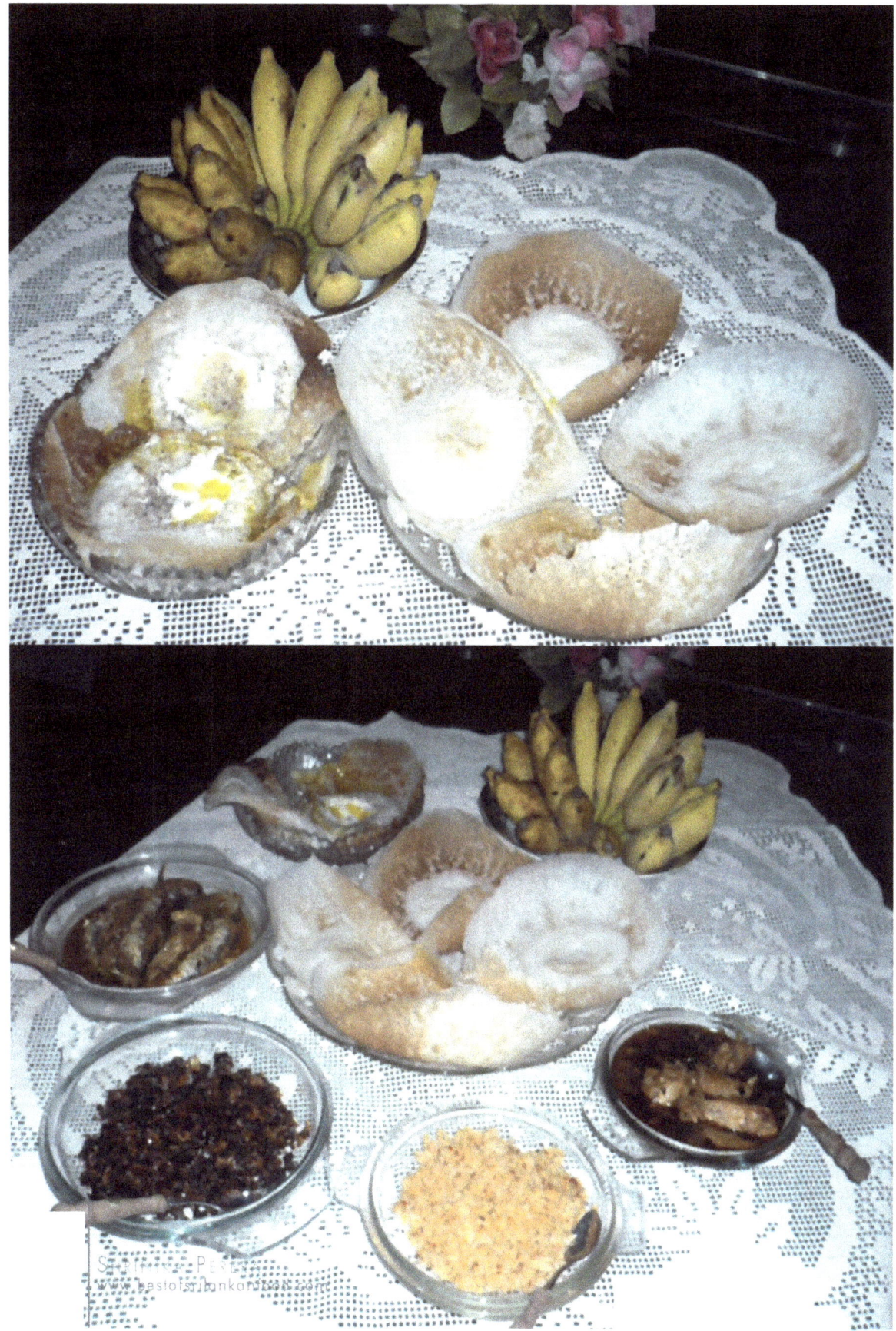

HOPPERS- (AAPPER)

Ingredients:

- 500g White /Red Rice flour or Chinese Rice Flour (available in Asian Super Markets)
- 2 tins Coconut cream or 4 cups thick coconut milk
- 2 tsp Sugar
- 2tsp Salt to taste
- 1 Egg or 1/2 tsp Bicarbonate of Soda
- 2 tsp Baking Powder or 2 tsp Yeast dissolved in 3 tbsps. of lukewarm water or 5 Tbsp. Coconut Toddy (please choose one option out of these 3 options.)

Method:

Sieve the flour into a bowl and add 2 tsp Baking powder (OR the dissolved yeast OR the coconut toddy) and mix well. Gradually add 2 cups of coconut milk mix and make a thick paste. Cover and leave for 6-8 hours. (If you are using coconut toddy, leave the mixture for 8-10 hours). After keeping for 6-8 hours, gradually add the balance thick coconut milk until the batter turns into a thin batter. Use only required and leave the excess milk aside to make the batter thin when necessary. Add salt, sugar, an egg, or bicarbonate soda to the paste and mix it into a thin batter. Leave the batter for further 15 minutes covered. Mix well. Ensure the batter is thin and runny. You can add more coconut milk if it's too thick. Heat a non-stick hopper pan, apply oil around it, and put a large spoon full or 3-4 tablespoons and turn around until batter sticks around the hopper pan. Cover and cook until it is crusty. Use a hopper spoon or a thin spoon and remove the hopper into a plate when the middle of the hopper is cooked.(2-3 minutes). If preferred, add a spoon full of the mixture, cover slightly, and add an egg into the middle before leaving for cooking, and you can make an egg hopper. Add pepper and salt for the egg before serving.

Serving Ideas: Meat /Fish curry/Prawns or chicken curry. Lunumiris, Pol Sambol, Seeni Sambol, Treacle, or Jaggery.

STRING HOPPERS

Utensils-String Hopper mats, String Hopper Mould, and a steamer.

Ingredients:

- 225g Roasted red /white rice flour (or Chinese Rice Flour)
- 1 tsp Salt to taste
- Boiling water to mix

Method:

Sift and place the roasted flour in a bowl. Add salt. Boil the water and set aside until the vapors are evaporated. Add the hot water to the flour little by little and mix until the mixture becomes a thick paste. Ensure the paste is not too hard or not too soft and doesn't stick in your hand. Don't over mix; it should be ready to use 3-4 minutes of mixing. Fill the mixture in a string hopper mold and squeeze out into string hopper mats in circular motion and steam for 8 to 10 minutes.

Serving Ideas: Serve with Coconut Sambal, Dhal Curry, Seeni Sambol, Kiri Hodi, Pol Mallun, or Meat/fish/chicken curry.

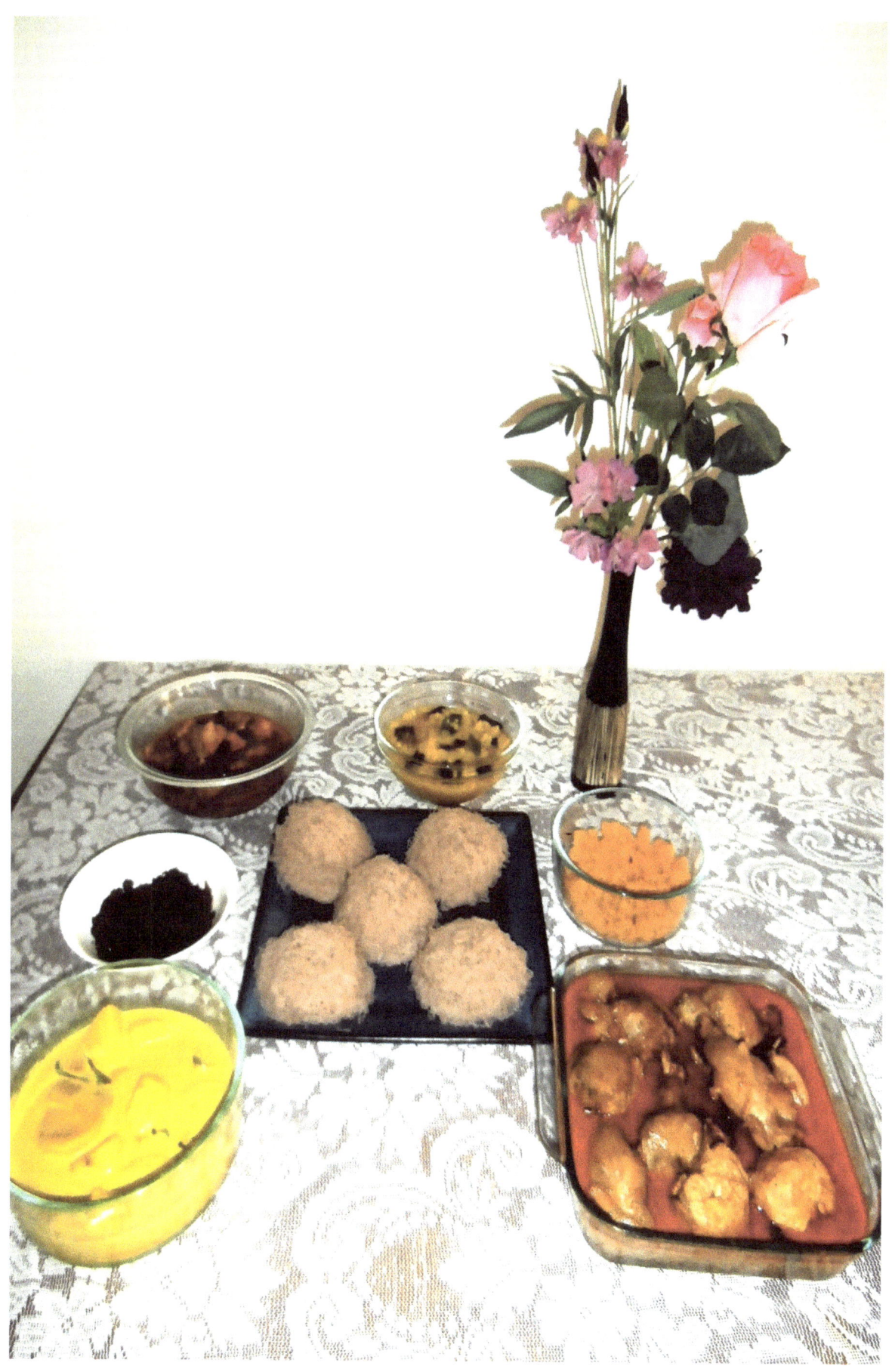

LUNUMIRIS

This is a very hot dish. It can be served with Roti, Milk Rice (Kiribath), Pittu, Hoppers, or Boiled Yam.

Ingredients:

- 5-6 Red shallots (or 1/2 Red Onion)
- 1tsp Peppercorn (Gammiris)
- 2 Cloves Garlic
- 1 tbsp. Flaked dried chilies
- 2Tbs Chili Powder
- 2tbs Maldivefish Flakes
- Few drops of lime juice.
- Salt to taste

Method:

Grind all ingredients to a paste, and add the lime juice. (When using chili powder, if you like mild flavor, use ½ tsp of chili powder. For medium flavor, use 1 tsp chili powder, and for hot flavor, use as per the recipe.)

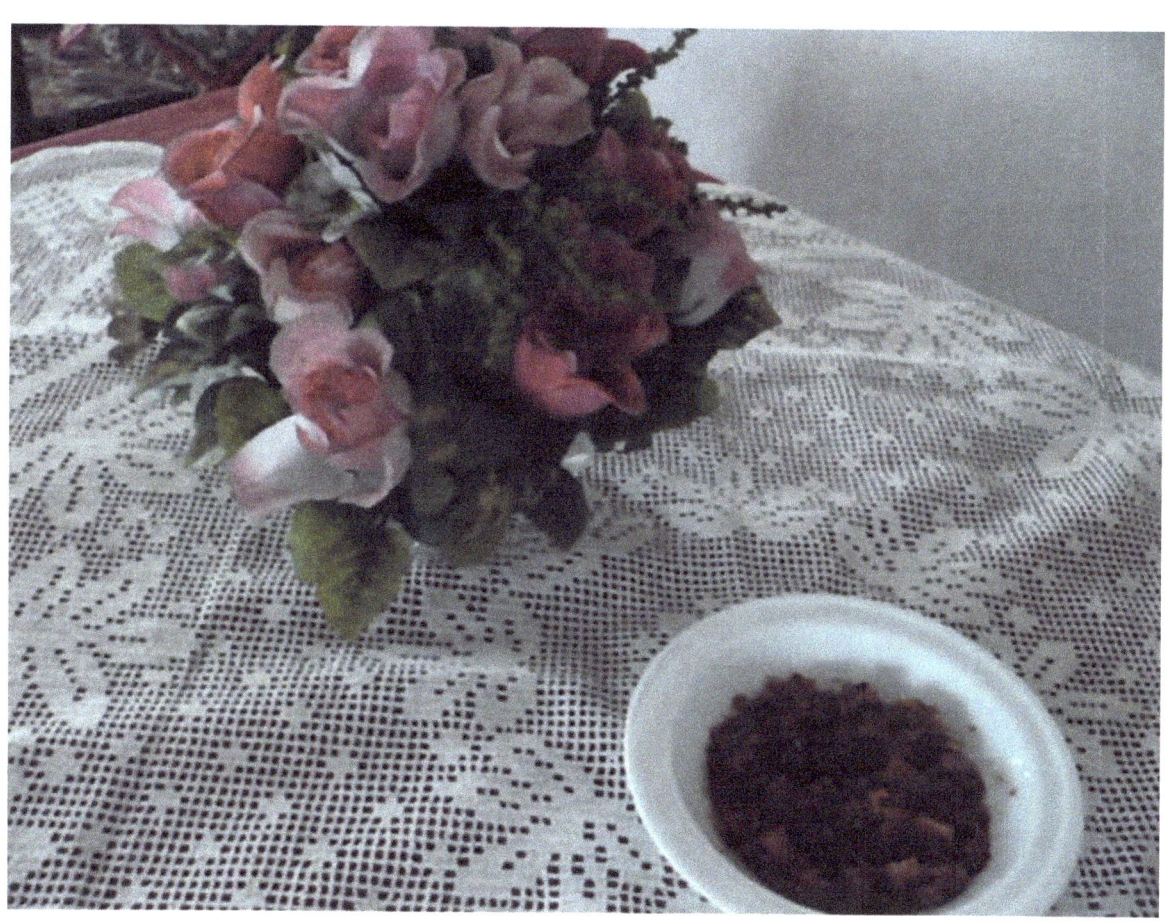

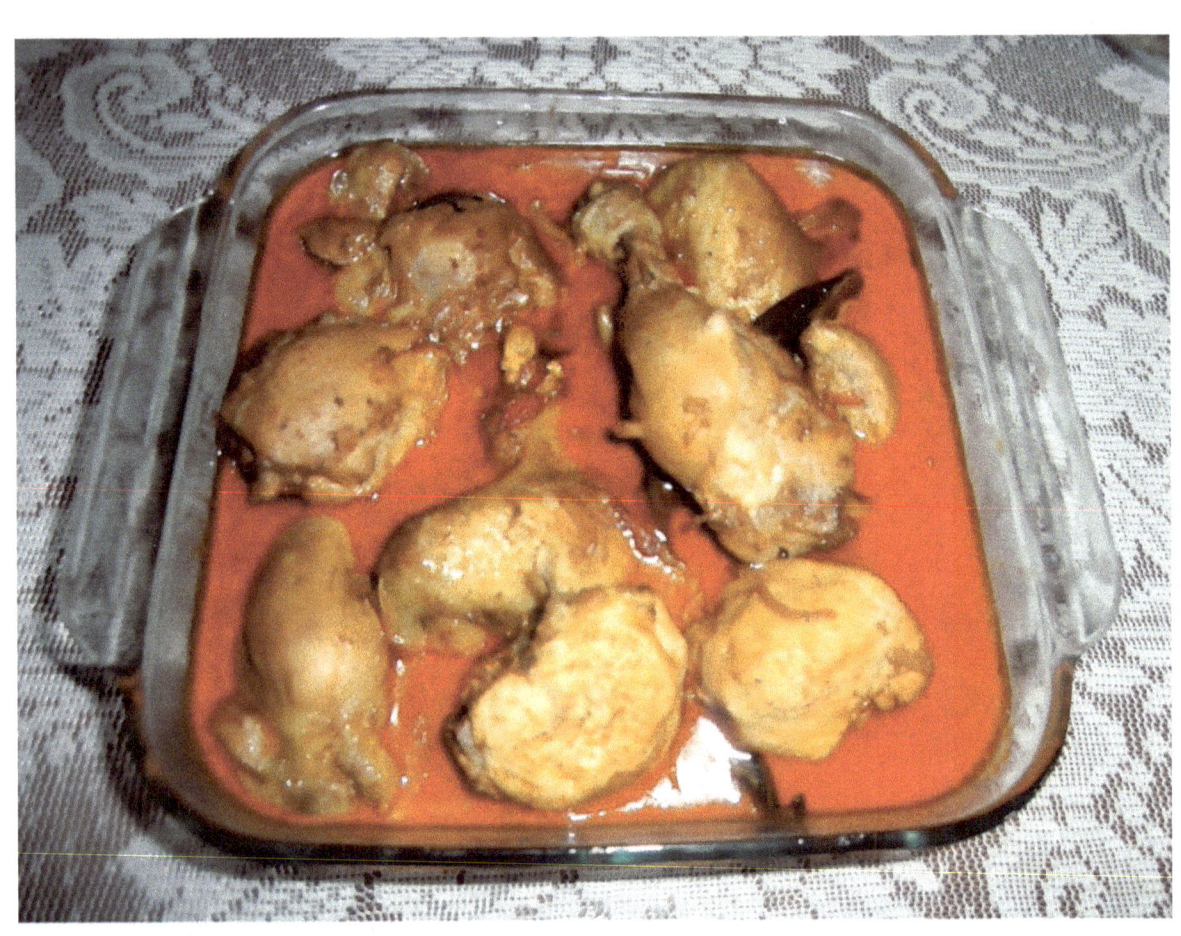

CHICKEN CURRY

Ingredients:

- 1 Whole Chicken
- ½ Large Onion- Chopped
- 1" piece Ginger- Grounded
- 3 Cloves Garlic- Grounded
- 2" stick Cinnamon
- 4" piece Rampe
- 1 Sprig Karapincha leaves
- 2 tsp Curry powder
- 4 tsp Chilli Powder
- 1/2 tsp Pepper Powder
- 8 Cardamom seeds- grounded (Karadhamungu)
- 8 Cloves-grounded (Karabu Nati)
- Salt to taste
- 1 cup Thick Coconut Milk
- 2 tbsp Coconut Oil

Method:

Heat oil in a pan and sauté chopped onions, green chilies, lemongrass, curry leaves, rampe, garlic, ginger, cardamom, and cloves. When onions are browned, add the pieces of chicken and fry on both sides. Add curry powder, chili powder, salt, pepper, and cinnamon and mix well. Cover and let the chicken pieces cook well. Simmer on low heat. When chicken is cooked, add thick coconut milk and cook on slow heat until the gravy is thickened and turns into a rich reddish-brown color.

(When using chili powder, if you like mild flavor, use ½ tsp of chili powder. For medium flavor, use 1 tsp chili powder, and for hot flavor, use as per the recipe. If you prefer mild curry, use sweet paprika to maintain a bright color and use turmeric for a beautiful golden-orange curry).

KIRI HODI

Ingredients:

- 1 cup Thick coconut milk
- 1 cup Water
- 1 Onion-chopped
- 2 Green chilies- Chopped
- 1" Piece Cinnamon
- 1 Sprig curry leaves
- ½ tsp Roasted Fenugreek seeds (Ulu hal)
- ½ tsp Turmeric
- ¼ tsp Curry powder
- Lime Juice
- Salt

Method:

Except for the lime juice and coconut milk, add all the other ingredients in a pan and bring to the boil and simmer for a few minutes. Add thick coconut milk and keep on stirring until the gravy is thick. Take off heat and add lime juice. Mix well.

Serve with String hoppers.

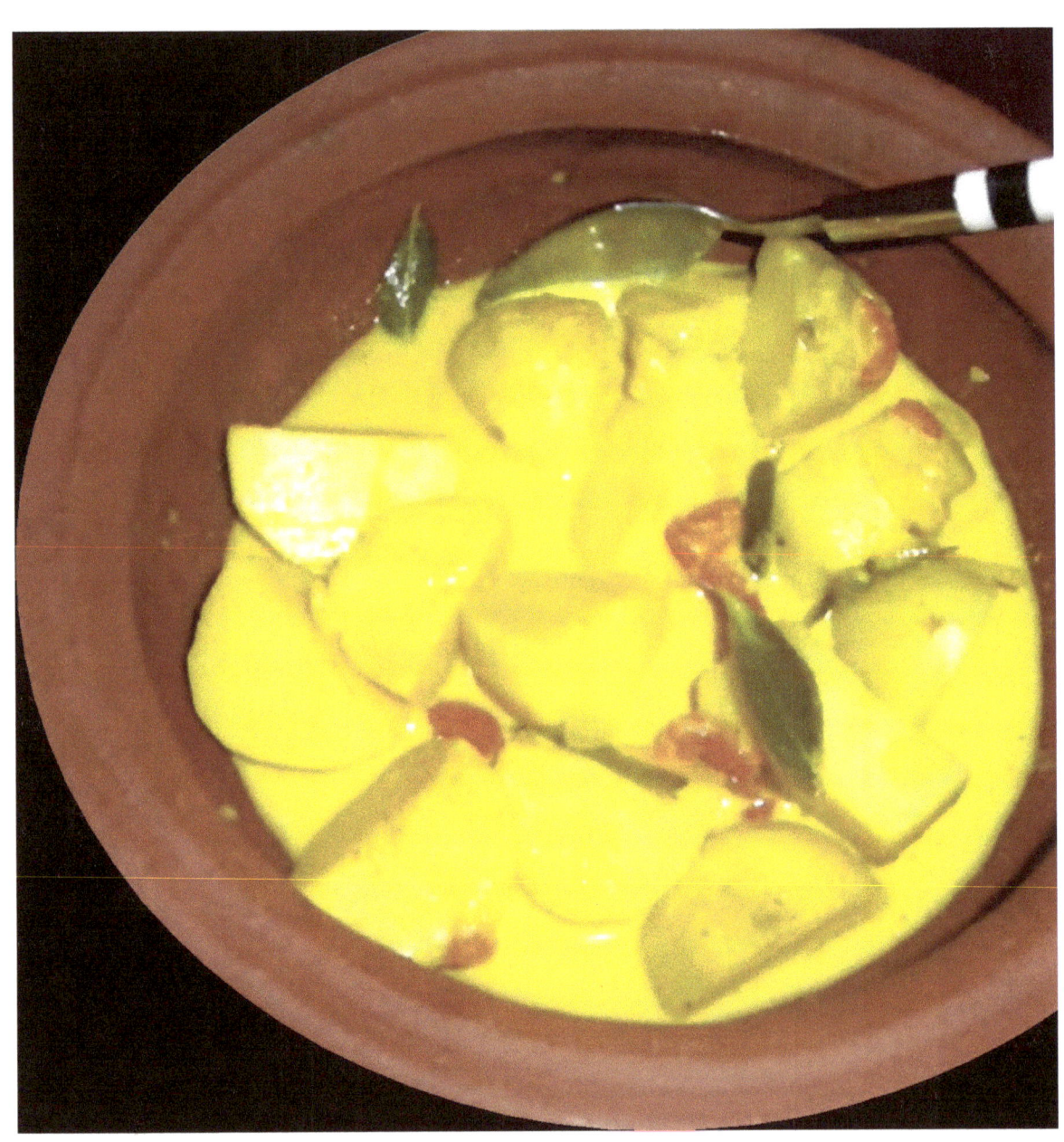

POTATO CURRY

Ingredients:

- 250g Potato
- ½ cup Thick coconut milk
- Water sufficient to cover the potatoes.
- ½ Small onion-chopped
- 1 Green chili- Chopped
- 1" Piece Cinnamon
- 1 Sprig curry leaves
- 1" Rampe
- ½ tsp Roasted Fenugreek seeds (Ulu hal)
- ½ tsp turmeric
- ¼ tsp curry powder
- Lime Juice
- Salt

Method:

Except for the lime juice and coconut milk, add all the other ingredients in a pan and bring to the boil and simmer for a few minutes until the potato is cooked. Add thick coconut milk and keep on stirring until the gravy is thick. Take off heat and add lime juice. Mix well. It could be served with string hoppers.

Serve with:

Hoppers, String Hoppers, Roti, Pitta, or Rice.

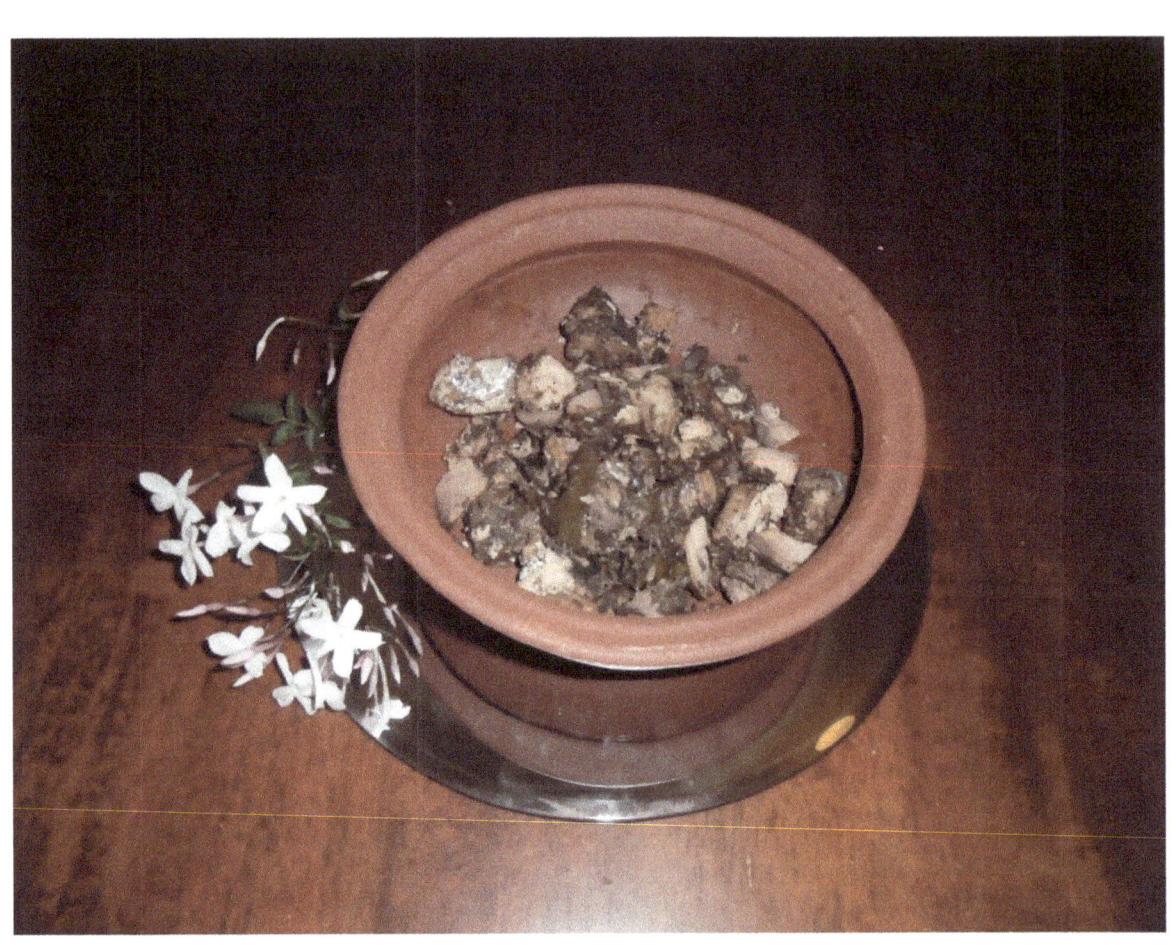

FISH AMBUL THIAL

Ingredients:

- 450g Fish (Red Fish)
- Pieces of Goraka –soak and grounded (Gamboge)
- 2 tbsp. Pepper Powder
- Chopped green chilies
- 3 Cloves Garlic chopped
- ½ tsp Ginger -Chopped
- Salt
- 1 Sprig Curry Leaves-Karapincha
- 2" Piece Rampe
- 2" Piece Cinnamon
- 1 tsp Chili Powder
- ½ cup water

Method:

Wash and cut fish into slices. Pat dry the fish and place in a saucepan. Ground all other ingredients into a paste and apply on the pieces of fish. Leave for 30 minutes. Add water and cover and cook on low heat until the fish is cooked in its own juice. Cook for 35 minutes on medium-low heat. Turn and mix the fish carefully until the liquid is absorbed. This curry could be kept for several days without refrigeration.

Serve with:

Pittu, Hoppers, String Hoppers, or Rice.

COCONUT SAMBAL

This is a very popular SriLankan food. It is usually called coconut sambal.

Ingredients:

1 Coconut scraped (or 1 Pkt Frozen scrapped coconut)

3 tsp Chilli Powder

1 tsp chili flakes or 2-3 dried chilies grounded

50g Red shallots or Onions

1 tsp Peppercorn (Gammiris)

2 Cloves Garlic

1/4 tsp Ginger

Salt to taste

3 tsp. Maldives Fish –Flaked (Optional)

1 sprig of Karapincha –Curry leaves

½ Lime Juice

Method:

Grind chilies, salt, onions, garlic, ginger, Karapincha (Curry Leaves), and Maldives fish into a thick paste, then add scraped coconut and grind all until all mixed together. Add ground pepper and ½ lime juice and mix well.

Serve with:

Hoppers, String Hoppers, or Rice

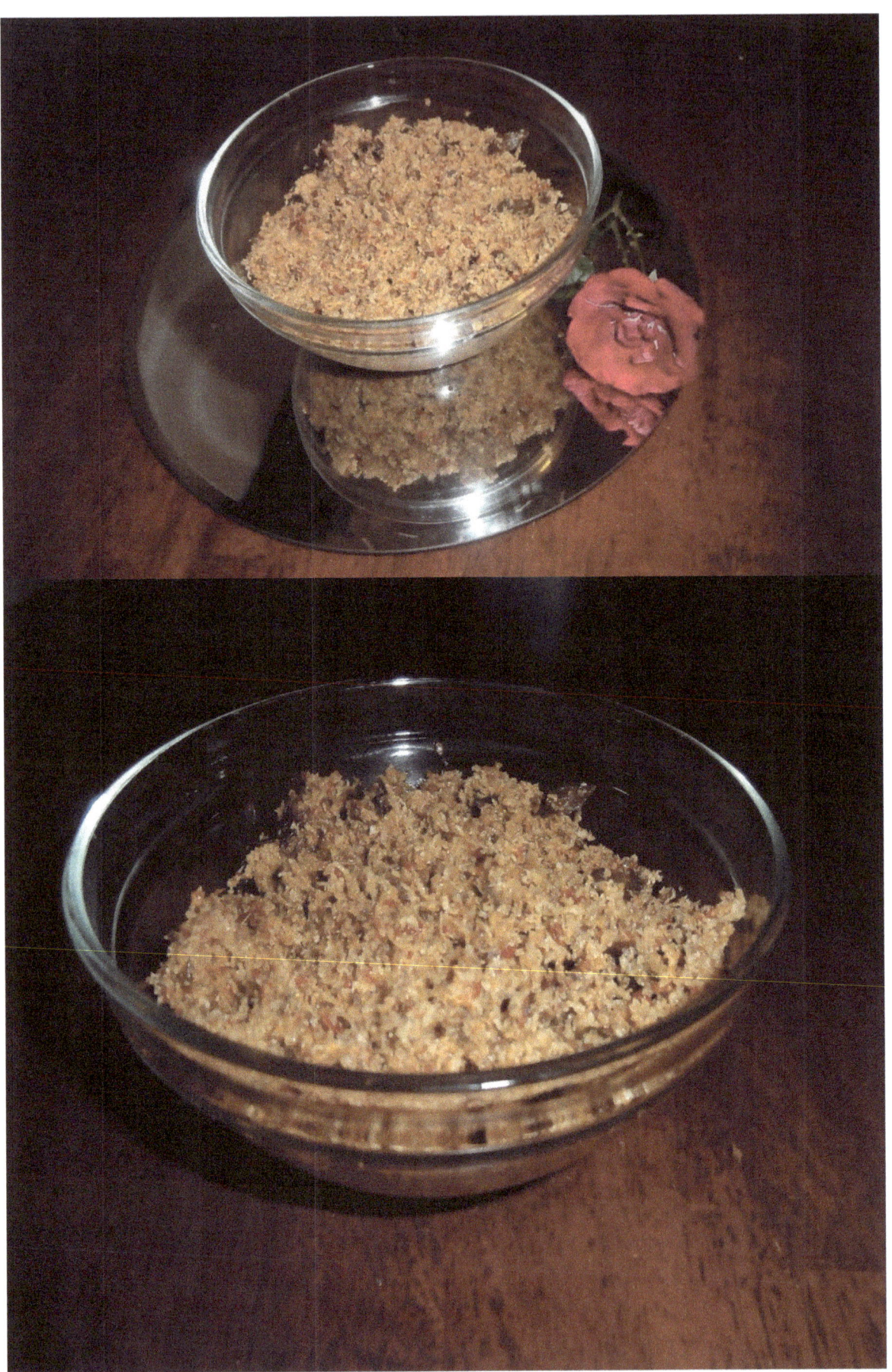

TEMPERED DHAL CURRY

Ingredients:

- 200g Dhal (Lentils –Red)
- 2 cloves garlic-chopped
- 1 Green chili- Chopped
- ½ Large Onion- Chopped
- 1 piece of cinnamon
- 1 Sprig Karapincha Leaves
- 1" piece of rampe
- ½ tsp Mustard seeds
- 3-4 Dried Chillies- broken into pieces
- ½ tsp turmeric
- ½ tsp chili powder
- 2 tbsp. Coconut Oil
- Salt
- ½ cup water
- 1 cup thick coconut milk

Method:

Wash and place the dhal in a pan and boil until the grains are cooked. Add oil into another pan, and once hot, add mustard seeds. When it's popped, add the Karapincha, rampe, onions, cinnamon, green chili, garlic, dried chili pieces, and once onions are brown in color, add the boiled dhal, turmeric, salt, chili powder, and saffron and add the 1 cup thick coconut milk and cook until the gravy is thick.

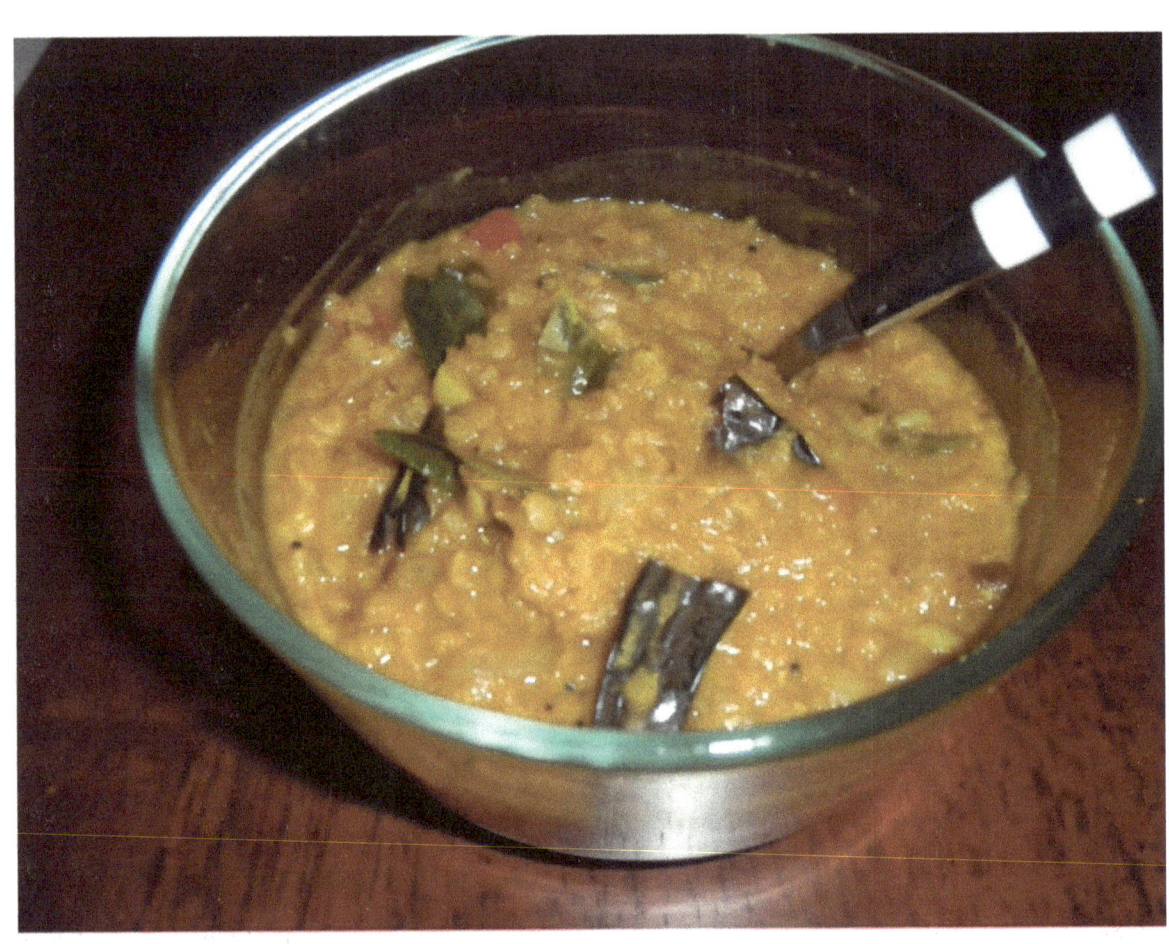

SEENI SAMBOL

Ingredients:

- 500g Onions- Chopped or sliced lengthwise
- 8 Cardamom seeds-grounded
- 8 Cloves-grounded
- 2" 2 Pieces of cinnamon
- A sprig of Karapincha Leaves Rampe
- 2" Stalk Sera (Lemon Grass)
- 1" Piece Ginger-Chopped
- 2 tbsp Chilli Powder
- 1 tsp Flaked Chilli Powder
- 1/2cup Thick coconut milk
- 1 Ripe tomato thinly sliced (Optional)
- 2 tbsp Tamarind Juice
- 1 tbsp Sugar
- Salt to taste
- 150g Maldive fish Flakes
- 4tb Coconut Oil

Method:

Heat Coconut oil in a pan and add chopped Onions, Rampe, Karapincha, sera, cardamoms, cloves, ginger, and cinnamon and fry until onions are golden brown.

Add chili powder, flaked chili powder, salt, sliced tomato, and Maldive fish and keep frying until the mixture is dry.

Squeeze tamarind into thick coconut milk and add to the mixture and lower the heat and cook until the moisture is absorbed.

Add sugar before taking off the heat and mix well. The sambal should be sightly moist. Remove lemongrass and the cinnamon stick before serving.

Serve with:

Hoppers, String Hoppers, Roti, Pittu, or Rice

(When using chili powder, if you like mild flavor, use ½ tsp of chili powder. For medium flavor, use 1 tsp chili powder, and for hot flavor, use as per the recipe.)

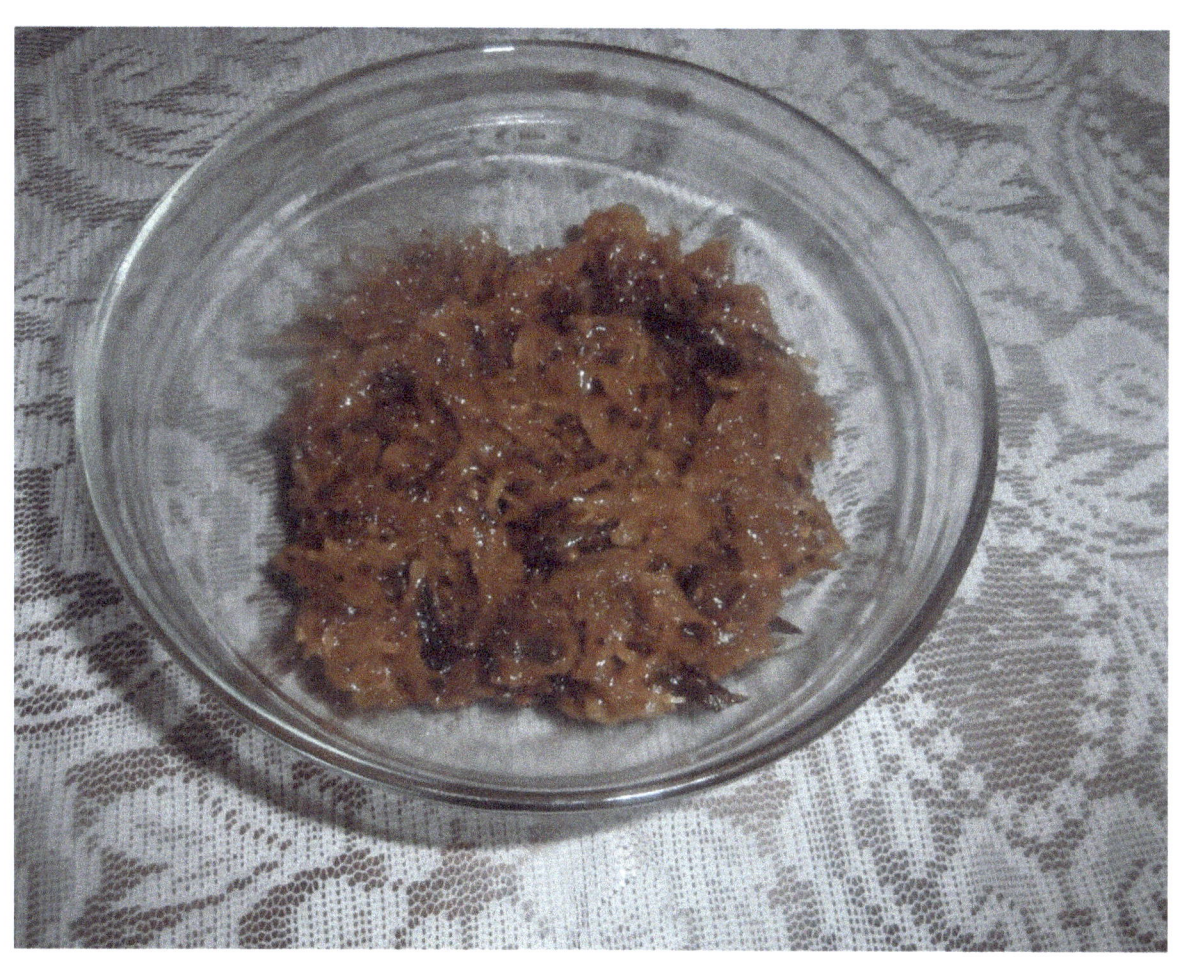

Rice

YELLOW RICE PILAU WITH CHICKEN

Ingredients:

- 250G Rice (Preferably Basmati Rice)
- 1 Big Onion chopped
- 1 Stick Cinnamon
- 1 Sprig of coriander leaves
- 1 Sprig Karapincha leaves
- 1 Cup Chicken stock
- 1 tsp Turmeric
- 2 tbs Butter
- 60g Sultanas
- Salt 4-5 Pepper
- 150G Boneless chicken
- Water to cook rice

Method:

Heat butter and fry the onion, karapincha, and chicken until golden brown. Add the rice, turmeric, cinnamon, salt, and pepper for 2-3 minutes. Add chicken stock and water. Mix well. Cover and simmer until rice is tender. Add coriander leaves and sultanas. Garnish with coriander leaves.

Serving Suggestions: Serve with:Chicken/ fish curry, Deval Prawns, Dhall Curry, Seeni Sambol, Salad, Boiled and fried eggs, Papadam.

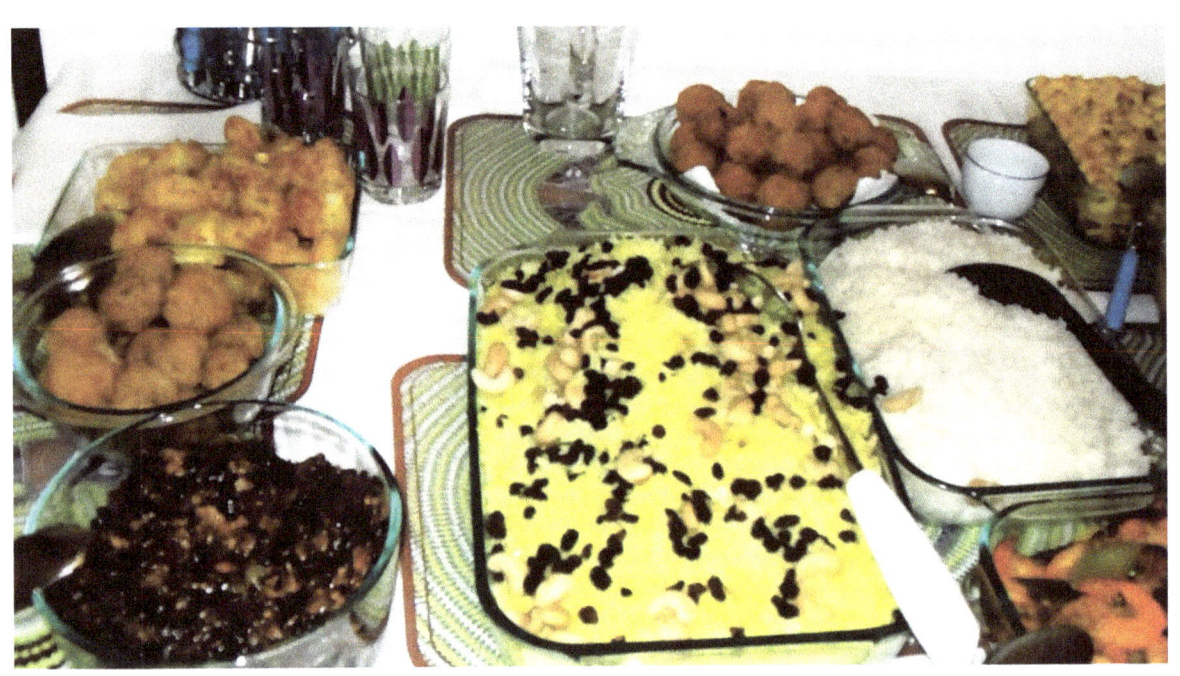

FRIED RICE

Ingredients:

- 2cups Basmati or Suduru Samba Rice
- 1 Large Onion –Sliced
- 5g Cashew- Fried
- 2g Sultanas- Fried
- 4 tbs Coconut Oil
- 1 Sprig Curry leaves –Karapincha
- 21" Rampe
- 8 Cloves
- 8 Cardamoms- Crushed
- 1 tsp Turmeric
- Coconut oil to deep fry

Method:

Deep fry Onion rings, Karapincha, and Cashew in coconut oil and leave aside. Wash and drain the rice. Heat coconut oil in a saucepan and fry chopped onions, Rampe, Cloves, Cardamom, Karapincha, and let the onions turn golden brown. Add the rice, salt ,water, and turmeric. Cover and cook at a moderate temperature for 15 to 20 minutes.Once the rice is cooked, remove all ingredients and serve in a dish decorated with the fried Onion rings, Fried Karapincha, Cashew, and Sultanas.

Serve with Chicken, fish, Deval Prawns, Dhall Curry, Seeni Sambol, Salad, Papadam, Eggs.

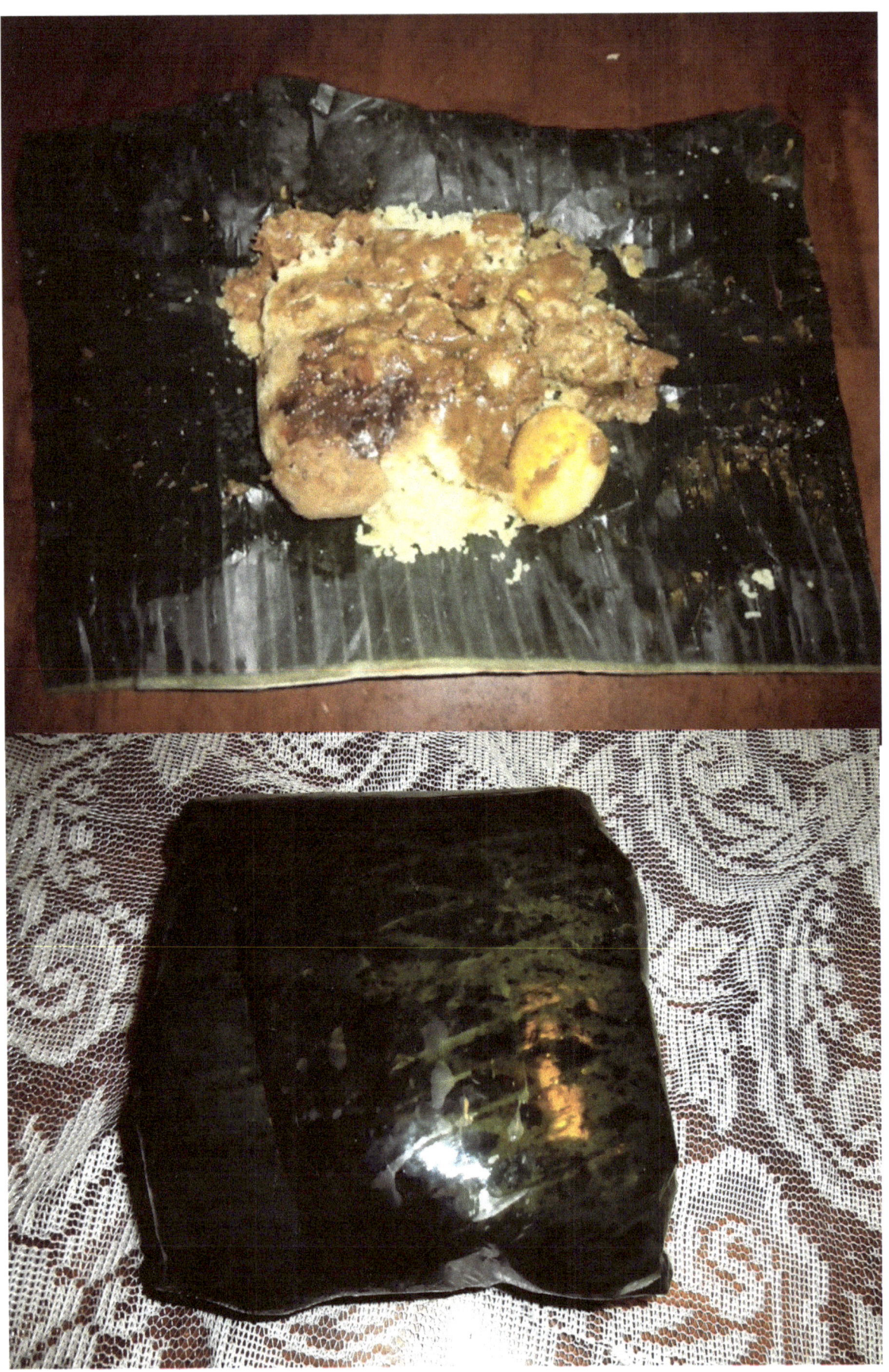

LUMP RICE

Menu

This is an ideal venue for a special occasion. Each lump of rice consists of Fragrant Rice, Chicken curry, a Cutlet, Brinjal Pahie, Seeni Sambol, Cashew Curry, and one hard-boiled egg deep-fried in oil. You can refer to the Curries and Salad recipes section.)

FRAGRANT RICE

Ingredients:

- 2 cups Basmati or Suduru Samba Rice
- 2 tbsp Coconut Oil
- 1 Medium Onion sliced
- 4 Cloves
- 4 Cardamoms
- ½ tsp Turmeric
- 3 cups Chicken stock
- Salt to taste

Method:

Wash and drain the rice and leave aside. Heat oil in a saucepan and fry onions till golden brown in color. Add other spices and rice frying well on moderate heat for few minutes. Add the stock, turmeric, and salt and bring to boil. Reduce heat to very low and slow cook for 15- 20 minutes covered with a lid. After the rice is cooked, gently fluff up the rice and remove all spices.

Serve hot with all the other curries wrapped in a banana leaf and oven-baked at 170-190c (350-375 f) for 15 to 20 minutes.

Curries and Salads

EGG SALAD

Ingredients:

- 250g Salad Leaves
- 100g cherry tomatoes- cut into halves
- 1 Cucumber chopped
- 1 Large onion cut into rings or half rings.
- 3 Green chilies cut diagonally
- 1 Lime juice
- 5 Eggs boiled
- 2-3tbs Salad dressing (1/2 cup Olive oil, 1 tsp mustard Cream, 1 tsp Vinegar, 1 clove garlic crushed, salt, and white pepper powder blended together)

Method:

Mix all ingredients together.

You can decorate this salad with boiled egg halves.

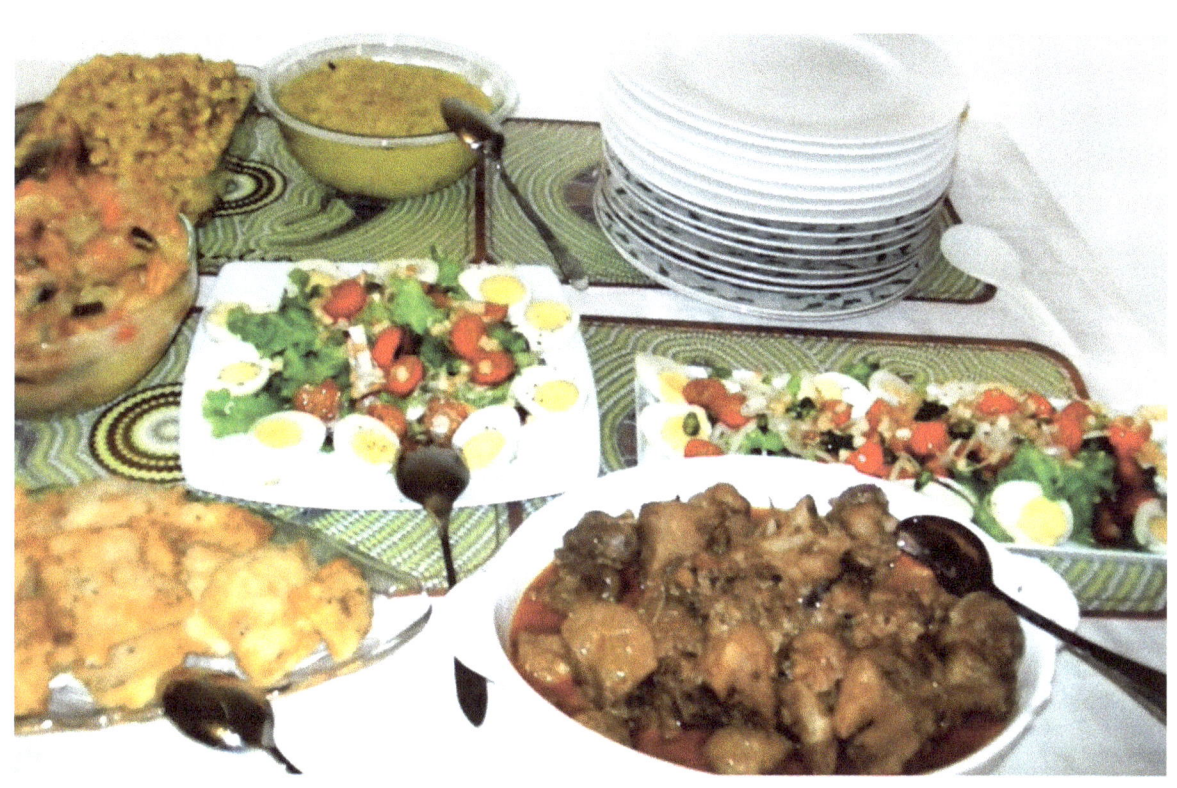

CUTLETS

Ingredients:

- 340g Salmon (or Boiled and minced Chicken or Beef)
- 340 g Potatoes
- ¼ tsp Cloves powder (Karabu nati)
- ½ Large onion chopped
- 2 Green chilies
- 2 Cloves garlic
- ½ tsp Ginger chopped
- 1 Sprig curry leaves- Karapincha
- 1 tsp Pepper
- Salt to taste
- 2 tsp Lemon to taste
- 2 tbs Coconut oil
- 100g Bread crumbs
- 1 Egg
- 1 liter Coconut Oil to fry

Method:

Boil and mash the potatoes. Heat the oil in a saucepan and gently fry onions , green chilies, garlic, ginger, curry leaves. Add Salmon (or boiled and Minced Chicken or Beef), pepper powder, salt and the boiled and mashed potatoes. Mix well. Take out from the heat and add lemon juice to taste. Set aside to cool. Shape into small balls about 1" in diameter. Dip into beaten eggs and coat with dry bread crumbs. Deep fry in coconut oil until golden brown in color. Drain on an oil - absorbent paper.

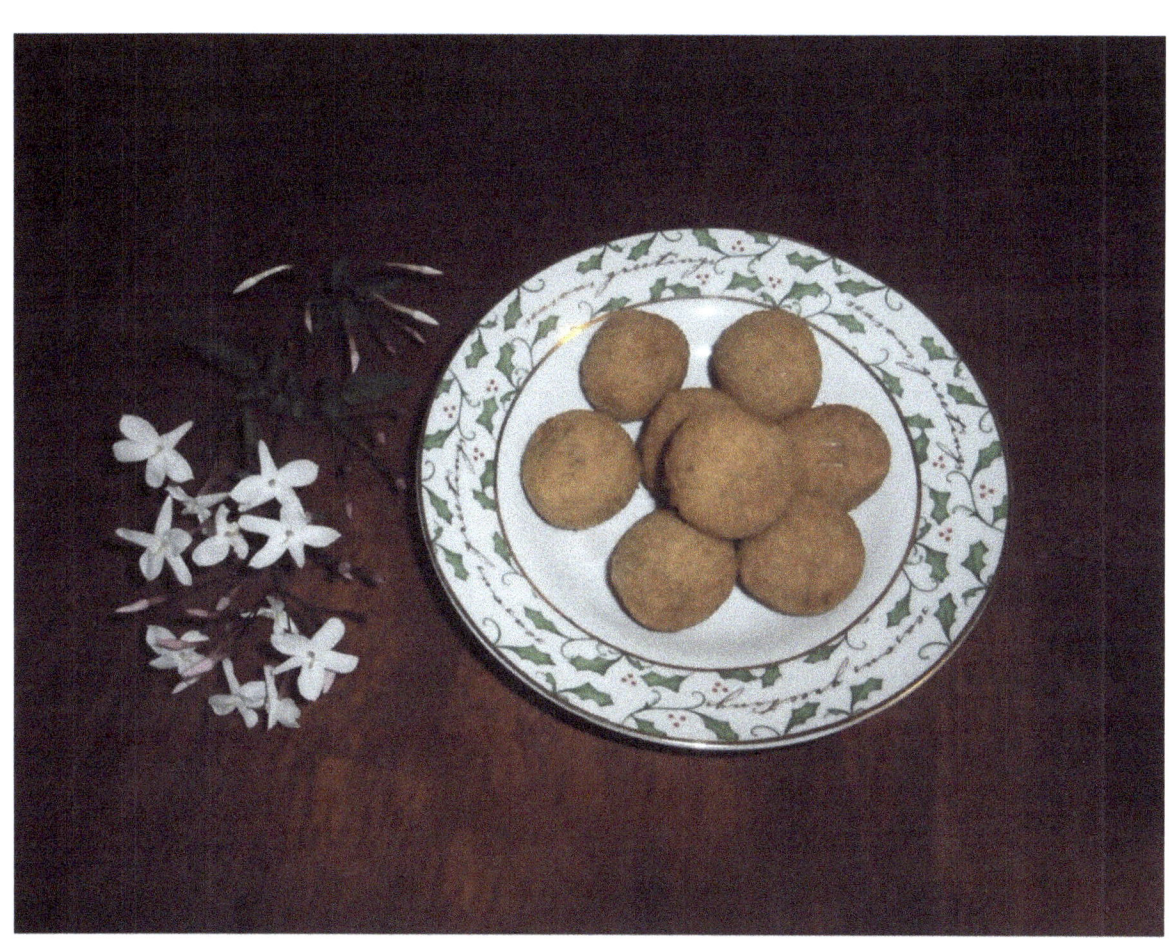

FRIED POTATOES

Ingredients:

- 250grams Potatoes
- 1 Large onion –sliced lengthwise
- 1 Sprig Curry leaves
- 2 Cloves of Garlic-chopped
- 2 Green chilies -chopped
- ¾ tsp Turmeric
- Salt to taste
- 1 ½ tsp chili flakes
- 2 tbsp Coconut Oil

Method:

Peel the skin of the potatoes and cut into 1-inch-thick pieces. Put the pieces in a saucepan and boil until the pieces are cooked. In a separate frying pan, heat Coconut oil and fry onions, chopped green chilies, and curry leaves. When onions are browned, add the boiled potatoes, turmeric, salt, and chili flakes. Mix well. If the texture of the tempered potatoes is dry, add few more drops of oil to get a rich wet texture.

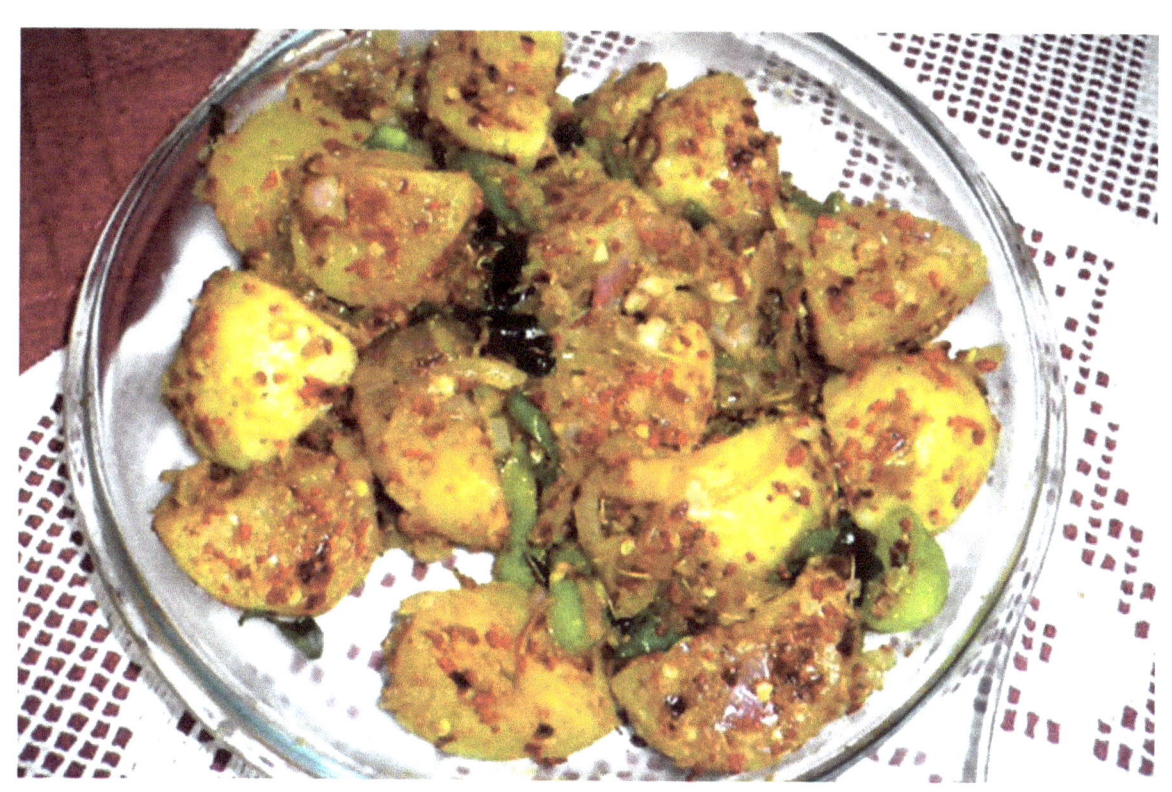

BEANS CURRY

Ingredients:

- 225g Green Beans
- ½ Large Onion-chopped
- 2 Green chilies -chopped
- 1 Sprig Karapincha (Curry leaves)
- 2 Cloves garlic
- 3/4 tsp Turmeric
- 1 1/2 tsp Curry powder
- ½ tsp Chili powder
- Few drops of lime juice
- 50 g Flaked Maldives fish
- Salt to taste
- ½ cup Coconut milk
- Coconut Oil to deep fry

Method:

Cut beans into 1" pieces or 1" strips. Heat Coconut oil and deep fry the beans until they are cooked and change to a dark green color. Deep fry the onions, green chilies, Karapincha, and chopped garlic. Take out onions and garlic when they are light brown in color. Add fried green beans, onions, green chilies, curry leaves, and garlic into a saucepan. Add turmeric, curry powder, and chili powder, salt, and Maldives fish and mix well. Add a ½ cup coconut milk and simmer until it forms into thick gravy.

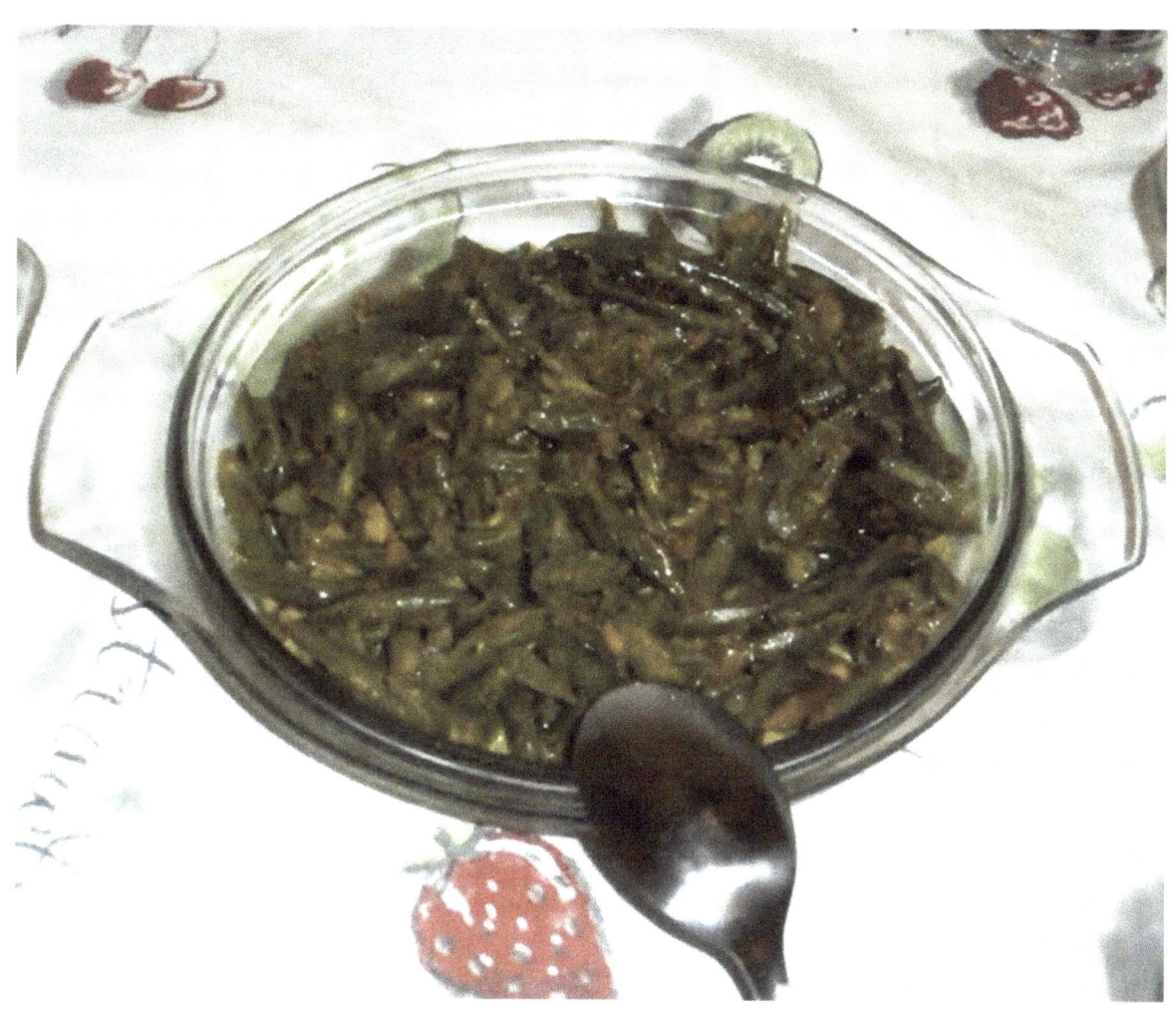

EGGPLANT MODJU/ WAMBATU MODJU

Ingredients:

- 300g Brinjals –(Eggplant, wambatu)
- 1 Large Onion- Sliced and cut into half rings
- 5 Green Chilies seeded and Chopped
- Salt and black pepper to taste
- 1 tbs Ginger grounded
- 1 tbs Garlic grounded
- 1 ltr Coconut oil for frying
- Salt to taste

Method:

Cut brinjals into thin strips about 2 ½ inches lengthwise. Mix with salt and leave for few minutes. Squeeze and deep fry in Coconut Oil until golden brown. Fry the half ringed onions, chili, ginger, and garlic for 2-3 minutes till soft. Then add the fried brinjals, salt to taste, and pepper. Cook for 3-4 minutes.

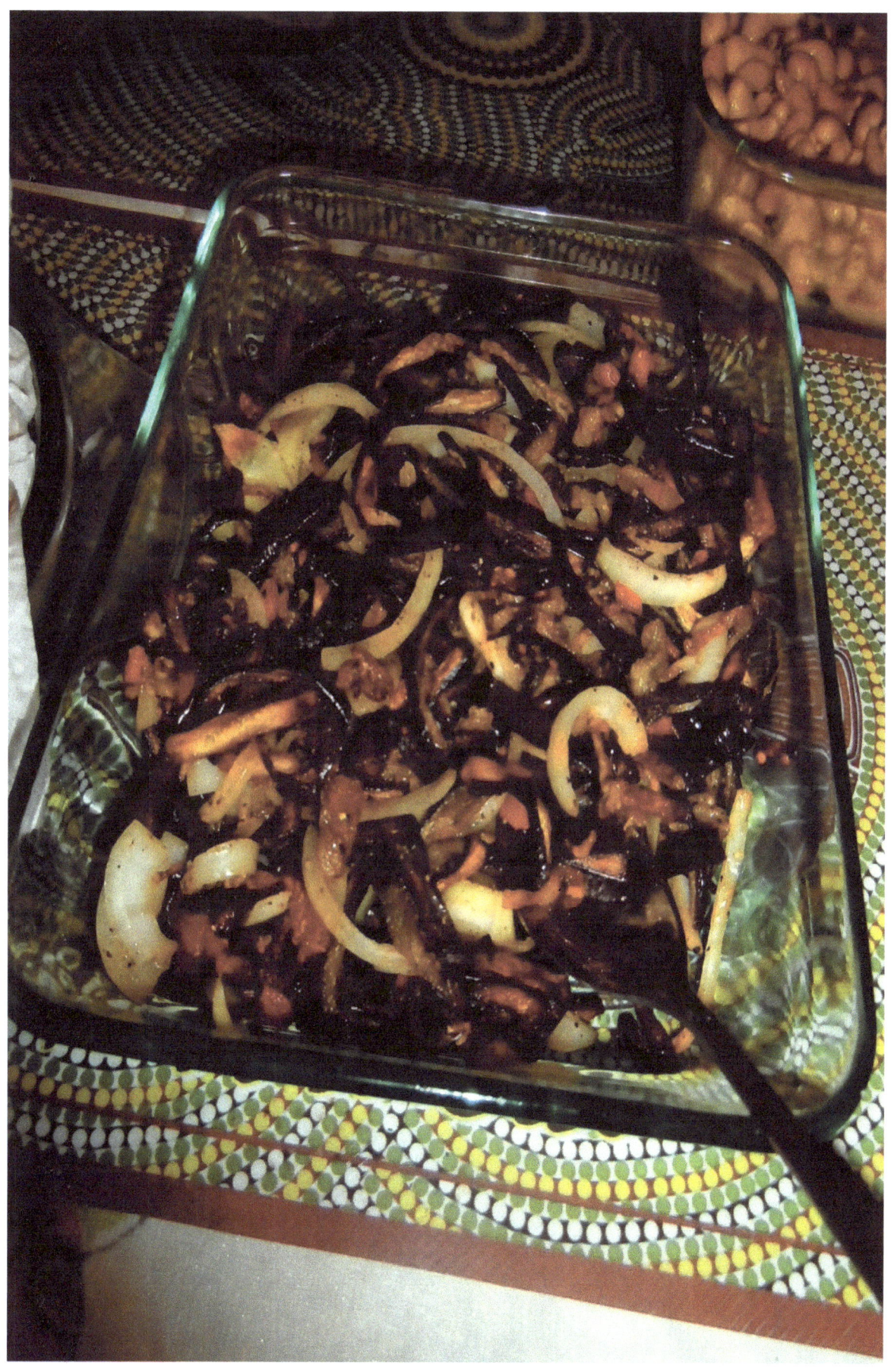

CASHEW CURRY

Ingredients:

- 250 g Raw Cashew
- ½ Small Onion- chopped
- 2 Green Chillies
- 2" Piece Cinnamon
- 1" Rampe
- 1 Sprig Curry leaves- Karapincha
- 1/2 tsp Turmeric
- 1 tsp Curry powder
- ½ tsp Chili powder
- 2 Cloves Garlic- chopped
- 2 Cups of water
- ½ cup Thick coconut milk
- 2 tbs Coconut Oil

Method:

Soak the cashew in water and leave for 2-3 hours or overnight to soften it. Add the soaked cashew into a saucepan of water and let it boil. Once the cashew is boiled, heat some coconut oil in a saucepan and fry the onions, garlic, curry leaves, rampe, cinnamon, and green chilies until the onions turn golden brown. Add the boiled cashew, turmeric, curry powder, salt, and chili powder and mix well. Add 1/2 cup thick coconut milk and simmer until it turns into a thick gravy.

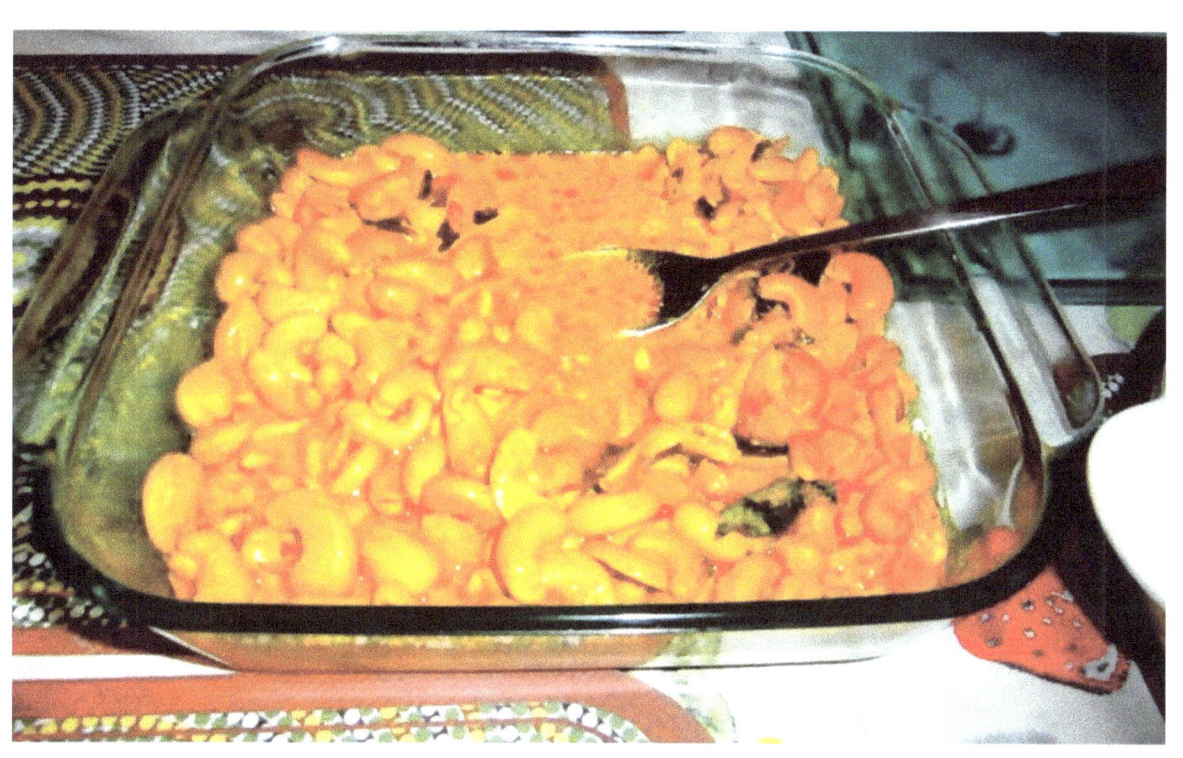

SINHALA ACHCHARU-PICKLE

Ingredients:

- 100g Capsicums
- 1 Small Raw Papaw- Cut into thin slices or 1" long thin strips
- 150g Long Beans (Maa Karal)- Ensure they are young and fresh, not overly mature. Cut into 1" long
- 100g Carrots- Cut into 1" long thin strips
- 200g Small Red Onions- Shallots
- 150g Green chilies- Lengthwise cut into 2 without separating from the stem.
- 2 tsp Grounded Mustard
- 1 cup Vinegar
- ½ inch Ginger-crushed
- 2 cloves Garlic-crushed
- ½ tsp Turmeric
- 2 tsp Pepper
- 2 tbsp Sugar
- Salt to taste

Method:

Heat the vinegar in a saucepan. Add green chilies, small red onions, carrot pieces, long beans, raw papaw pieces, garlic, and ginger and simmer for a few minutes. Finally, add the capsicums. Leave for 2 minutes and take out from the heat. Add mustard, turmeric, pepper, sugar, salt, and mix well. Store it in a tight clean bottle and refrigerate.

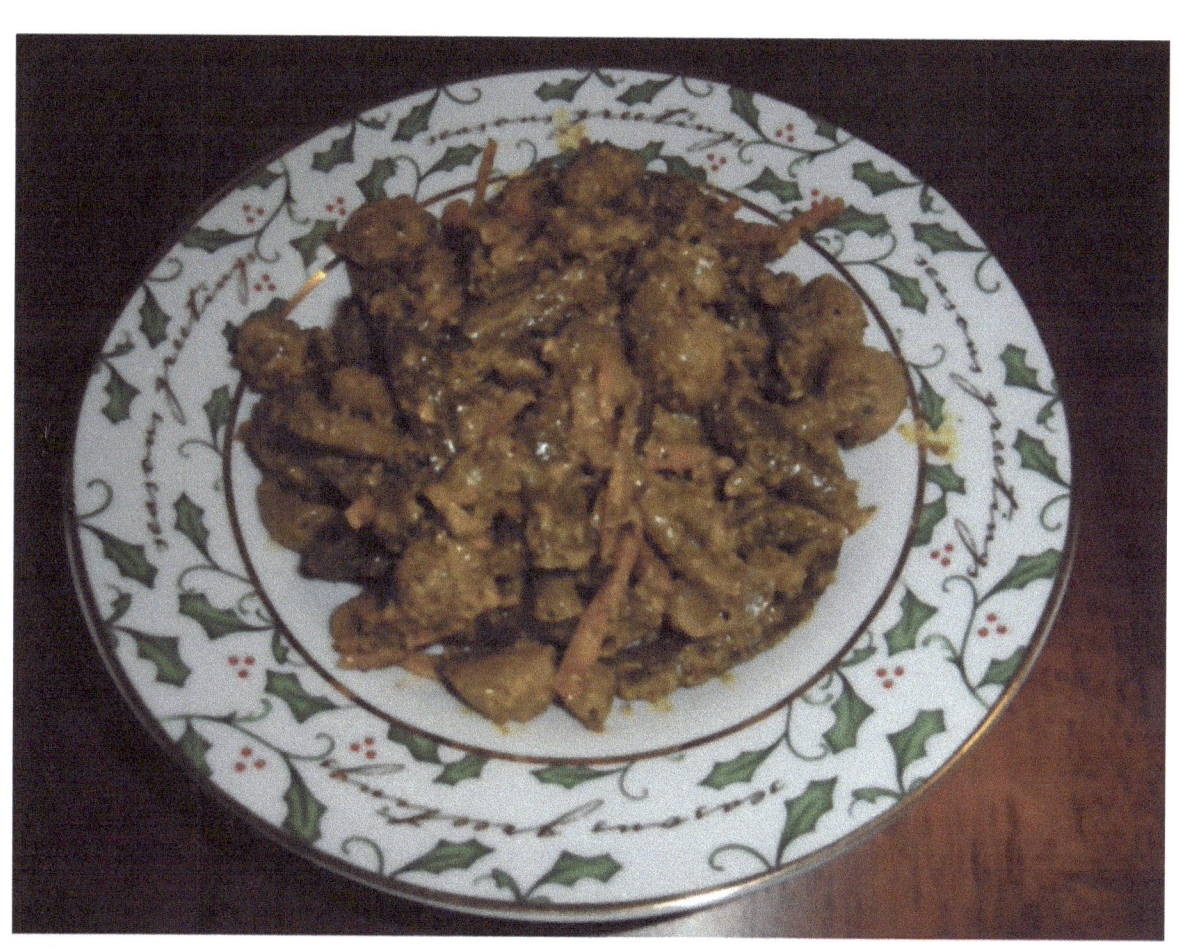

PINEAPPLE CURRY

Ingredients:

- 1 Small ripe Pineapple or a tin of pineapple chunks
- 1 tsp Chili Powder
- 1 tsp Curry powder
- 1 Sprig curry leaf-Karapincha
- 2" Cinnamon
- ½ Onion- chopped
- 2 Green chilies- chopped
- 1/2tsp Turmeric
- 1" Rampe
- 2 Cloves Garlic- chopped
- ½ cup Thick coconut milk
- 2 tbs Coconut Oil

Method:

Cut the pineapple into ½" pieces. Heat some coconut oil add the onions, green chilies, cinnamon , garlic, and leave let the onions turn golden brown. Add the pineapple, spices, and salt and mix well. Cover and let it cook in the pineapple juice for a while, then add the coconut milk, mix it and let it simmer for a thick curry on low heat.

(When using chili powder if you like mild flavors, use ½ tsp of chili powder. For medium flavors, use 1 tsp chili powder, and for hot flavor, use as per the recipe. If you prefer mild curry, use sweet paprika to maintain a bright color and use turmeric for a beautiful golden-orange curry).

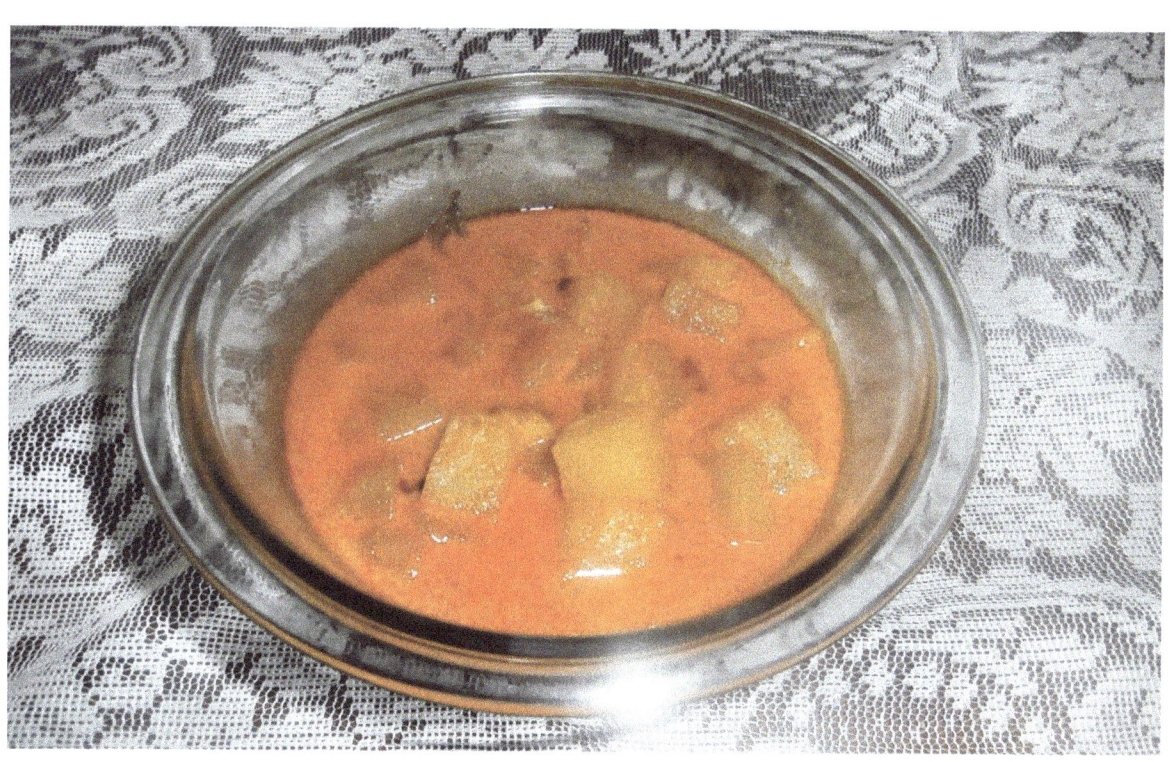

POLLOS CURRY

Ingredients:

- 250g Young jack
- ½ Large Onion-chopped
- 2 Green chilies chopped
- 1 Sprig of curry leaf –Karapincha
- 5 Cardamoms- crushed
- 5 Cloves- crushed
- 2 Cloves Garlic- chopped
- 1 tsp Ginger
- 1/2tsp Pepper
- 1-2 pieces Goraka
- 2" Cinnamon
- 2 1/2 tsp Chilli Powder
- 1 tsp Curry powder
- 2 tbs Coconut Oil
- ½ Cup Thick Coconut milk

Method:

Cut the young jack into 1" long and ¼" thick pieces and boil until the pieces are cooked. Remove from the heat without over boiling. In a fresh saucepan, fry the onions, green chilies, garlic, curry leaves, and ginger with 2 tbsp. coconut oil and add the boiled young jack once the onions are browned. Add all the remaining spices and mix well. Add ½ cup thick coconut milk and simmer until it turns into a thick reddish-brown curry.

(When using chili powder, if you like mild flavor, use ½ tsp of chili powder. For medium flavor, use 1 tsp chili powder, and for hot flavor, use as per the recipe. If you prefer mild curry, use sweet paprika to maintain a bright color and use turmeric for a beautiful golden-orange curry).

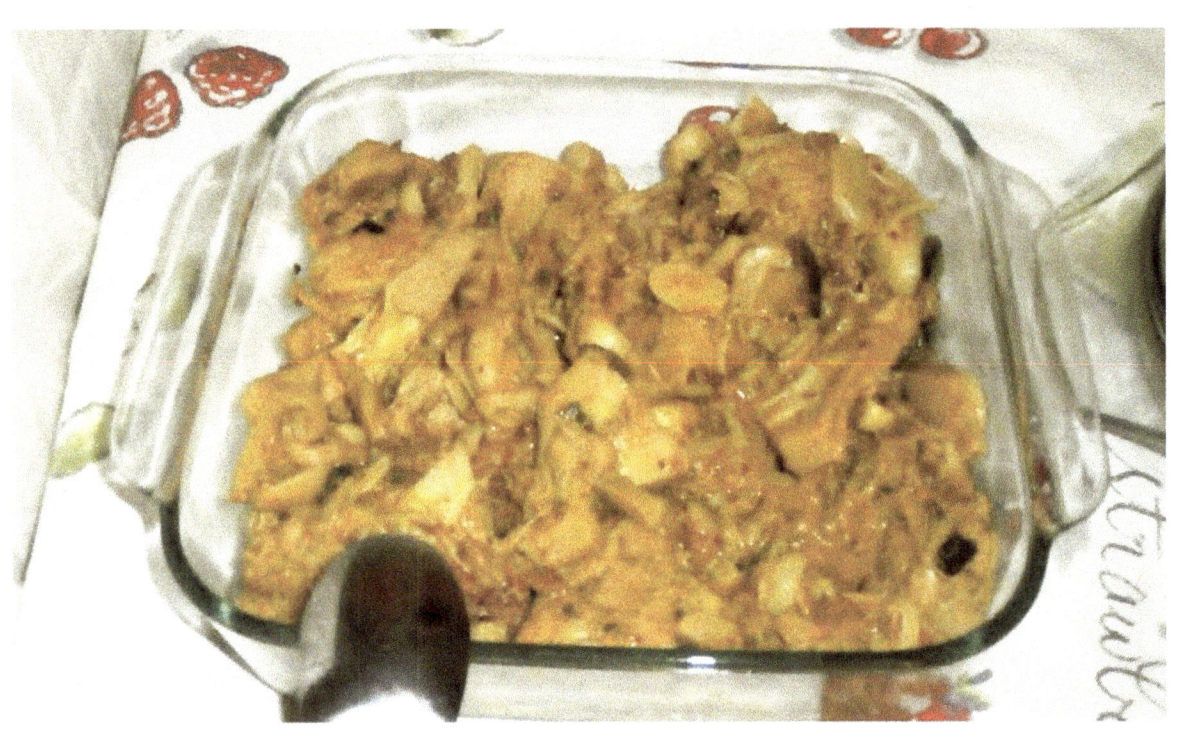

FRIED DHAMBALA CURRY

Ingredients:

- 200g Dambala
- ½ Large onion- chopped
- ½ Large Tomato- chopped
- 2 tsp Curry Powder
- 1 tsp Turmeric
- 1 1/2tsp Chili powder
- 2 Green chilies chopped
- ½ tbs Maldive fish
- 2 Cloves Garlic
- 1 Sprig Curry leaf- Karapincha
- ½ cup Thick Coconut milk
- 1" Cinnamon Piece
- 2 tbs Coconut Oil

Method:

Wash and cut Dambala into slices. Deep fry them for 2-3 minutes. In a separate saucepan, heat some coconut oil and fry onions, rampe, karapincha, green chilies, cinnamon, and garlic. When the onion is browned, add the curry powder, chili powder, turmeric, salt, and tomatoes. Let the tomatoes fry, then add the thick coconut milk, and when the curry is boiling, add the fried dambala. Simmer until it turns into a thick gravy.

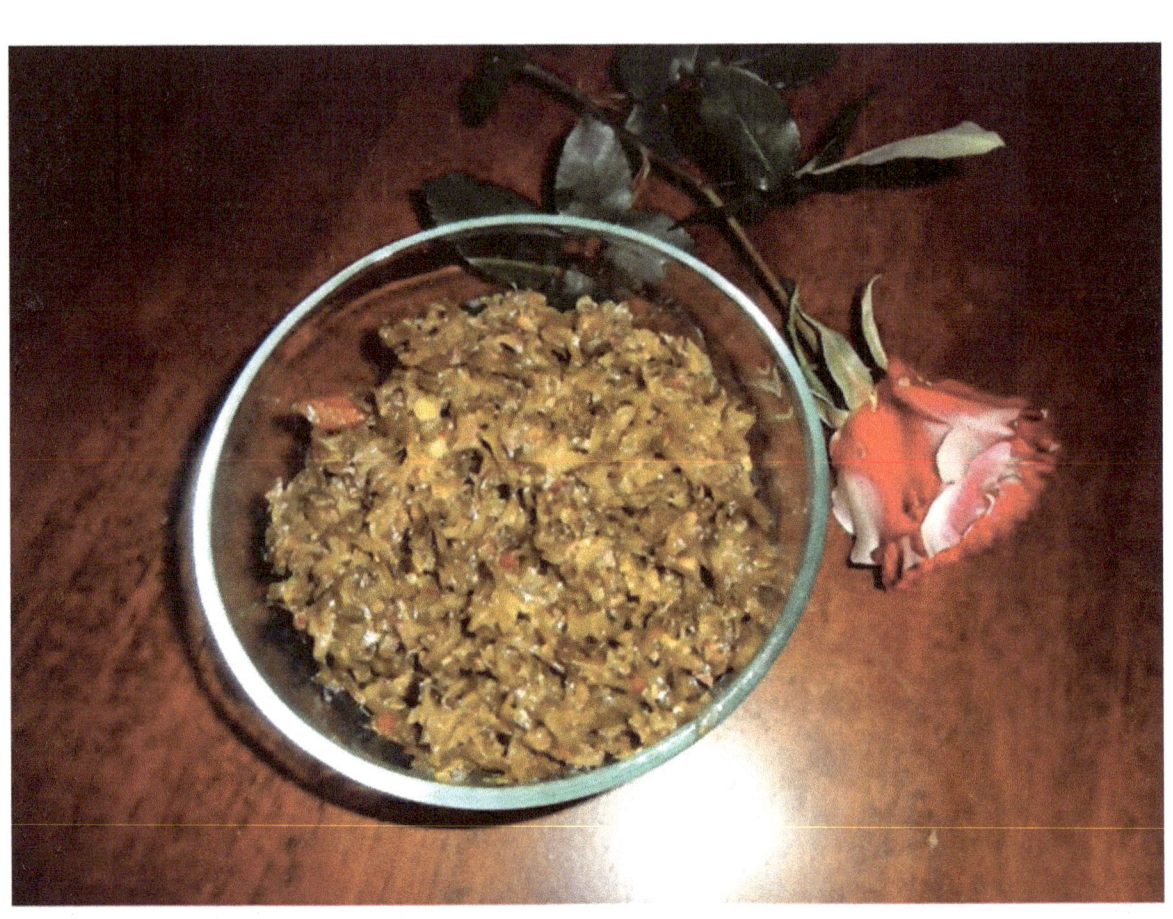

BRINJAL PAHIE

Ingredients:

- 250g Brinjals –(Eggplant, wambatu)
- 1 Large Onion- Sliced and cut into half rings
- 5 Green Chilies- seeded and chopped
- 3 tbs Mustard paste/cream
- 2 tbsp Sugar
- ½ cup Coconut Vinegar
- ½ tsp Turmeric powder
- Salt and black pepper to taste
- 1 tbs Ginger grounded
- 1 tbs Garlic grounded
- 3 Tomato wedges
- 1 tbs Corriander
- 1 tbs Cumin powder
- 1 tsp Chilli powder
- 1" Cinnamon stick
- 1 tbs Taramind pulp
- 1 cup water
- 1 ltr Coconut Oil for frying
- Salt to taste

Method:

Cut brinjals into thin strips about 2 ½" lengthwise. Mix with salt and safran and leave for a few minutes. Squeeze and deep fry coconut oil until golden brown. Blend the mustard cream, vinegar, ginger, garlic, and turmeric pulp along with the water and blend into a smooth paste. Fry the half ringed onions, chili, tomato, and cinnamon for 2-3 minutes till soft. Then add the blended mixture and the rest of the ground spices. Add sugar and cook for 3-4 minutes and finally add the fried brinjals. Stir well cover and simmer for 15 minutes. Season with salt and black pepper.

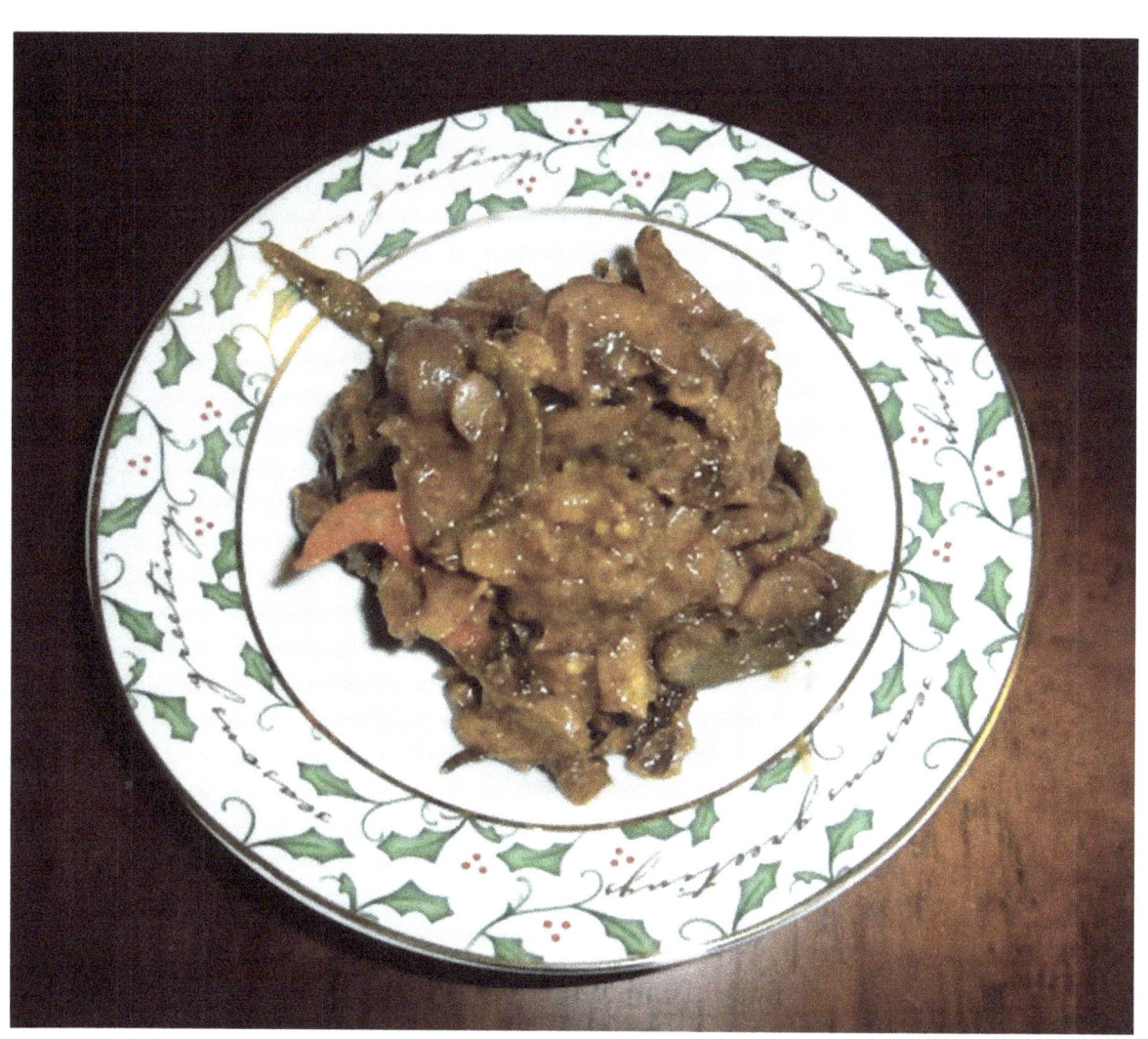

PUMPKIN WITH ROASTED COCONUT CURRY

Ingredients:

- 400 g Pumpkin
- 4 Tbsp. Scraped Coconut
- 2 Tbsp. Raw Rice –Washed
- 2 Tsp Mustard Seeds
- 4 Cloves Garlic
- ½ Onion Chopped
- 1 Green Chilli
- 1 Tsp Turmeric
- 1 Tbsp. Maldive Fish
- 1 ½ Cups Mild Coconut Milk
- 1 Cup Thick Coconut Milk
- 1 Spring Curry Leaves
- 1 Piece Rampe
- 1" Piece Cinnamon
- Salt to taste
- ¼ Tsp Pepper Powder

Method:

Heat a pan and add mustard seeds, then add the coconut and raw rice, and pan-fry until the coconuts and rice turn to golden brown. Once golden brown, take out from the heat and grind it into a paste with the garlic and set aside.

Cut the pumpkin into ½" to 1" long pieces. Cover and boil the pumpkin in a pan with 1 ½ cup water, chopped onions, green chilies, saffron, cinnamon, karapincha, and pepper for 10-15 minutes. Mix the grounded garlic and coconut paste into 1 cup thick coconut milk and add the mixture to the boiled pumpkin. Add the Maldive fish and salt to taste and simmer for 2-3 minutes.

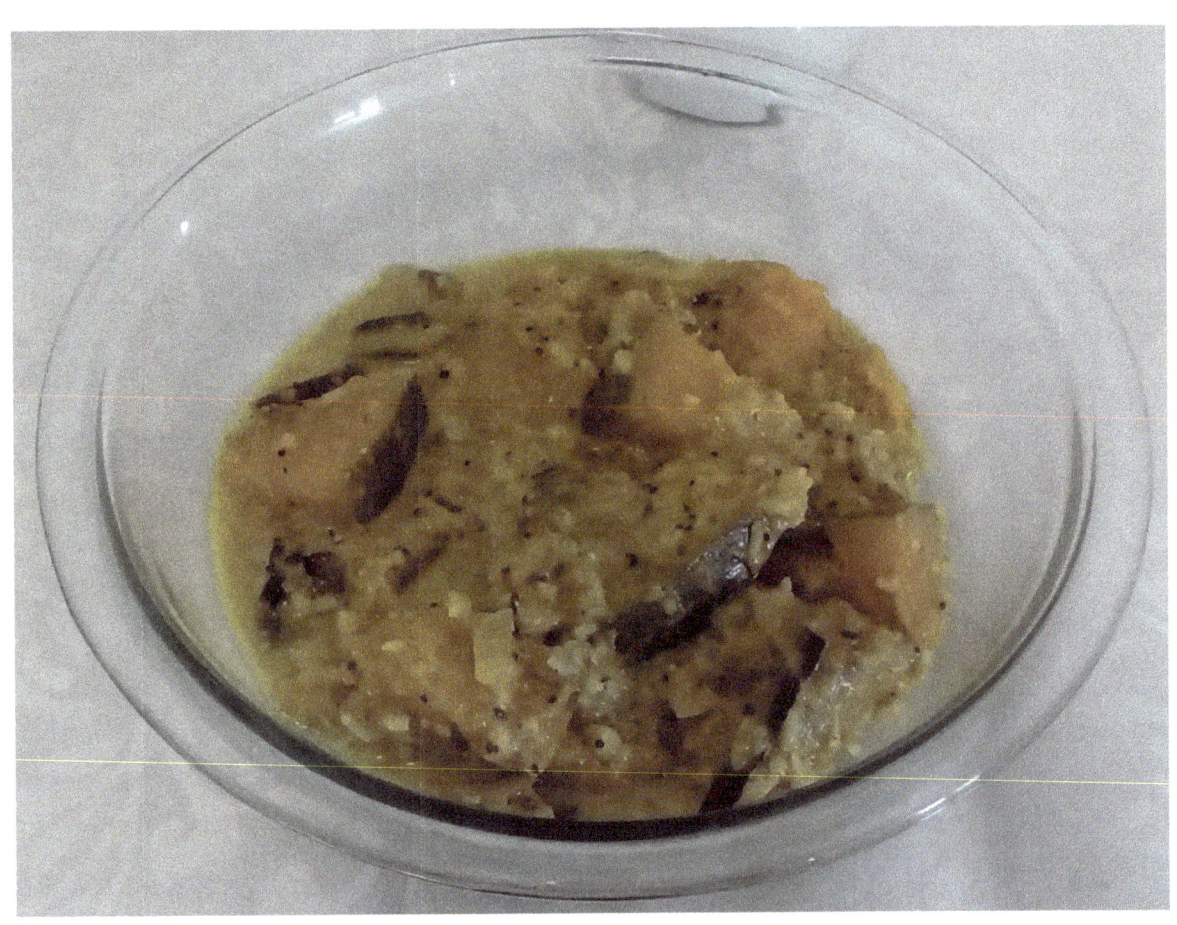

Seafood and Fish

DEVILLED PRAWNS

Ingredients:

- 500g Prawns -Cleaned
- 2 medium Onions- quartered
- 50g Small red Onions
- 2 Capsicums –Cut into angle wise large Cubes-Red or Green
- 4Tbs Tomato paste
- 30g Tomatoes -Chopped
- 40g Leeks - Cut into angle wise large pieces
- ½ tbsp. Flaked Chilli pieces
- 2 tbs Coconut Oil
- ½ tsp Turmeric
- 1 Tsp chopped Garlic
- 1 Tsp. Chopped Ginger
- 5 Green chilies- Lengthwise cut into four
- 1 Lime Juice
- Salt to taste
- 1 Sprig curry leaf-Karapincha,
- 2" Rampe
- 1" Cinnamon

Method:

Wash and clean the prawns. Add salt, saffron, and lime juice and leave aside. Heat some coconut oil in a separate pan and when the oil is hot, add chopped onions, Karapincha, Chopped ginger, and garlic and let the onions turn to a golden color. Add flaked chilies and small onions. Let it fry for further 1-2 minutes. Then add the prawns, capsicums, green chilies and let it fry for 3-4 minutes. Then add the leeks and the tomato sauce. Mix well and add lime juice and tomato pieces. Remove the deval from heat before the tomato is cooked.

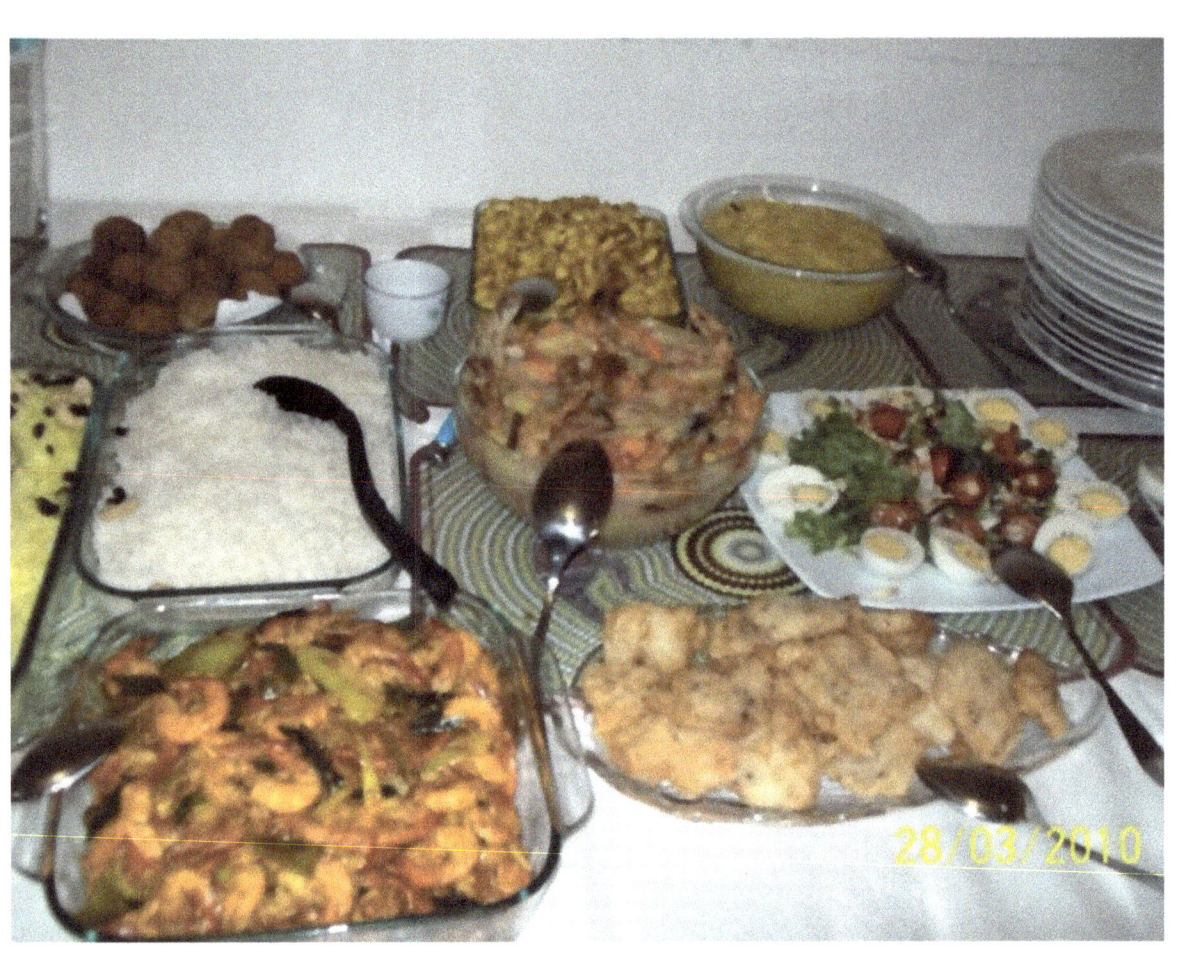

FRIED FISH

Ingredients:

- 250g Fish
- 1 Lime juice
- Salt to taste
- 1 cup Corn Flour
- Coconut Oil to fry

Method:

Cut into 1 ½" long pieces. Add salt and lemon juice. Leave for 15 minutes. Coat with cornflour and deep fry until it turns a golden brown color.

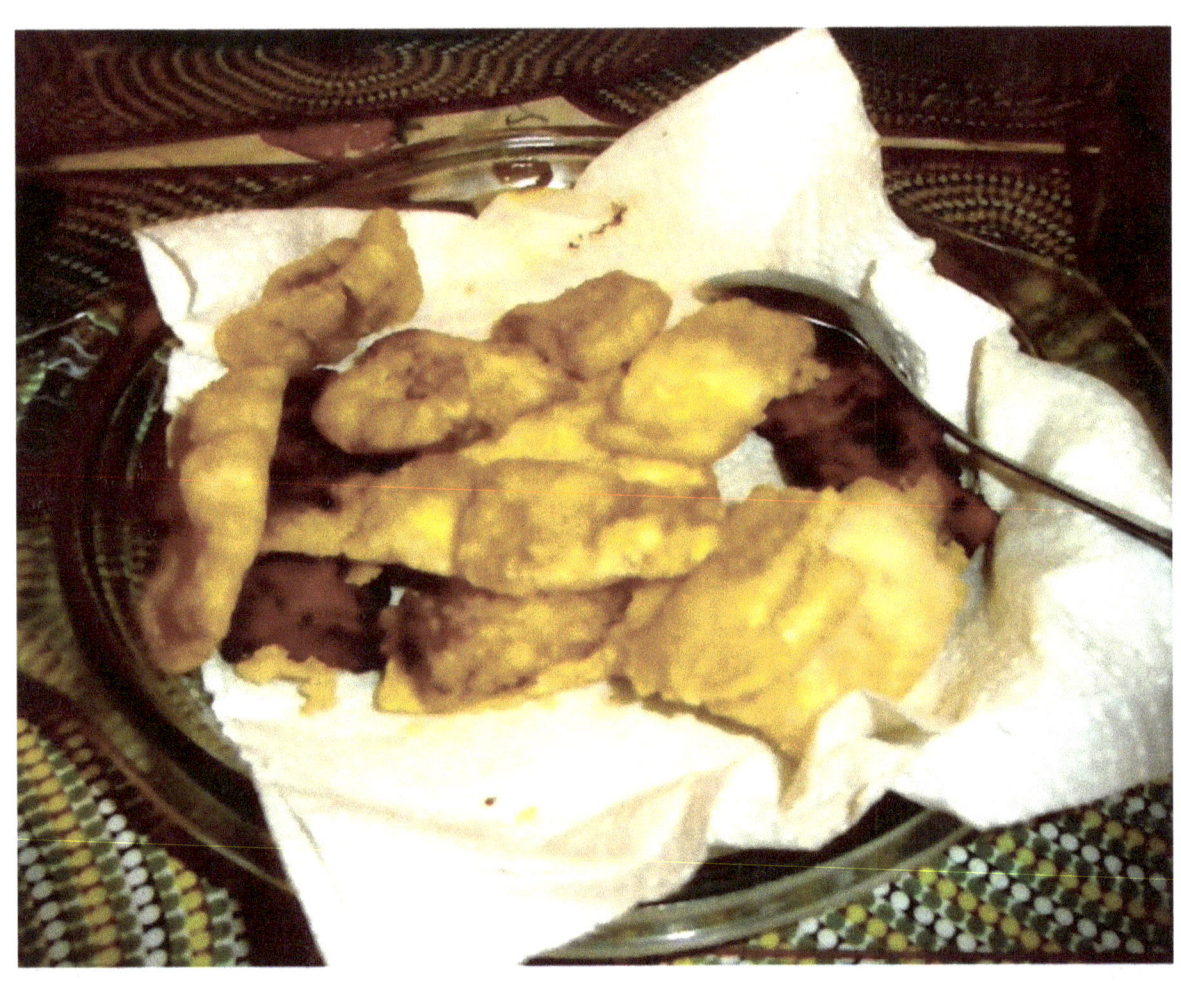

PRAWNS CURRY

Ingredients:

- 250g Prawns
- ½ Onion chopped
- ½ Tomato Chopped
- ½ tbsp Flaked Chili pieces
- 2 tsp Chili powder
- 1 tsp Curry powder
- 2 tbs Coconut Oil
- 1/2 tsp Turmeric
- 1 tsp Chopped Garlic
- ½ tbsps Chopped Ginger
- 2 Green chilies- Chopped
- Juice from 1 Lime
- Salt to taste
- 1 Sprig curry leaf-Karapincha,
- 2" Rampe
- 1" Cinnamon
- 1 cup Water
- ½ cup Thick coconut milk
- Chopped Coriander leaves
- 1 Tomato Chopped
- 1/2 tsp Coriander seeds - ground

Method:

Clean and wash the prawns. Heat some coconut oil in a saucepan and fry chopped onions, curry leaves, garlic, ginger, and cinnamon pieces. When the onions are golden brown, add flaked chili flakes, turmeric, salt, chili powder, and curry powder, and add the prawns and mix well and cook for few minutes with lid covered until the prawns are cooked. Then add water and let the prawns cook on moderate heat and add tomatoes. Then add the thick coconut milk, tomatoes, and grounded coriander seeds and simmer under low heat until the curry is thick red golden brown in color. Garnish with chopped coriander leaves.

(When using chili powder, if you like mild flavor, use ½ tsp of chili powder. For medium flavor, use 1 tsp chili powder, and for hot flavors, use as per the recipe.)

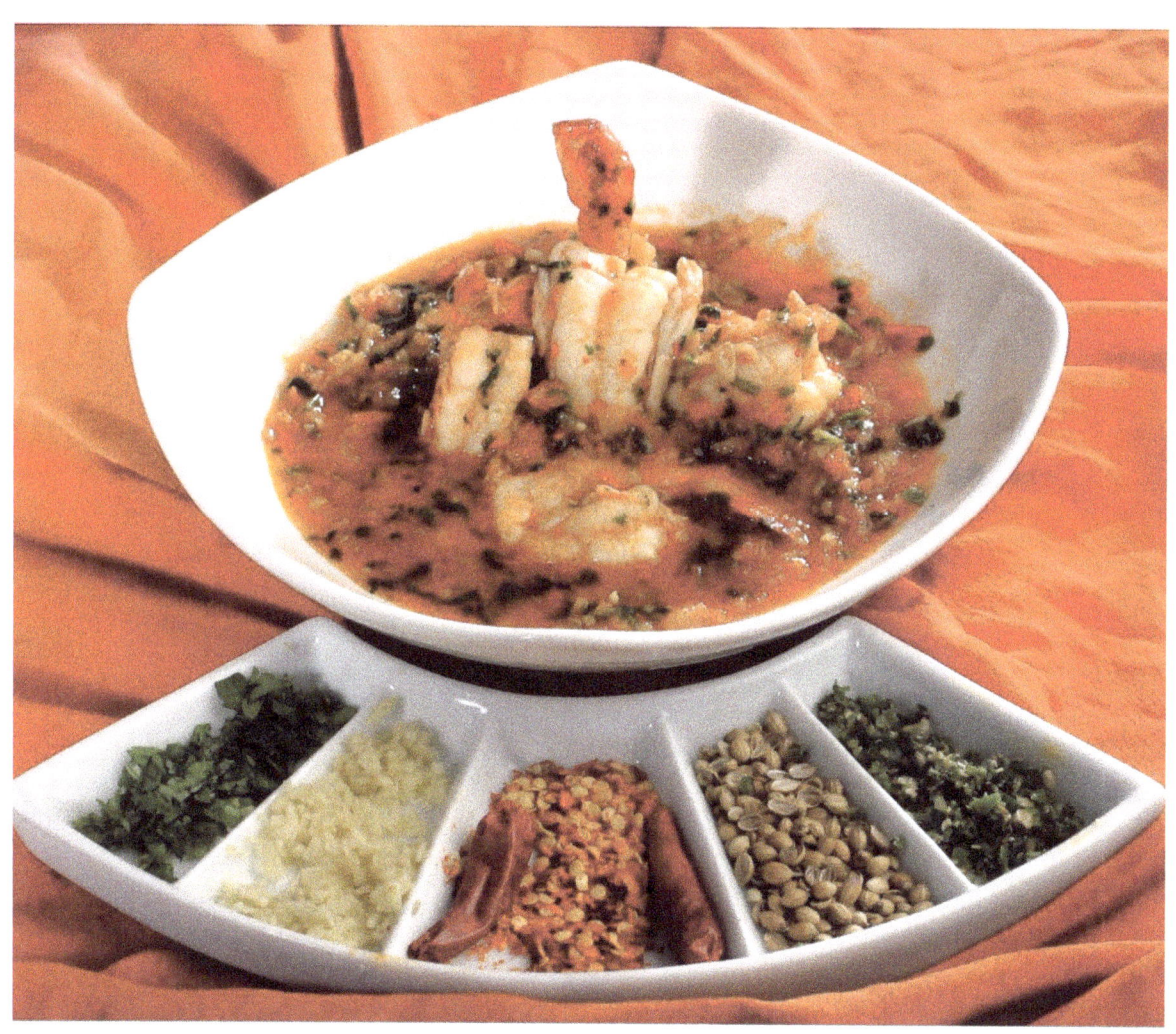

CRAB CURRY

Ingredients:

- 4 Crabs
- ½ onion- chopped
- ½ tbsp. Flaked Chili pieces
- 2 tsp Chili powder
- 1 tsp Curry powder
- 2 Tbs Oil
- 1/2 tsp Turmeric
- 1 Tsp chopped Garlic
- ½ tbsp chopped Ginger
- 2 Green chilies- Chopped
- Juice of 1 Lime
- Salt to taste
- 1 Sprig curry leaf-Karapincha,
- 2" Rampe
- 1" Cinnamon
- 2 cups water
- ½ cup thick coconut milk
- Chopped Coriander leaves

Method:

Clean and wash the crabs. Cut each crab into four pieces. Chop the 2 main large claws. Heat some coconut oil in a saucepan and fry chopped onions, curry leaves, garlic, ginger, and cinnamon pieces. When the onions are golden brown, add flaked chili pieces, turmeric, salt, chili powder, and curry powder. Then add the crabs and mix well and cook for a few minutes. Then add water and let the crabs cook on moderate heat. Then add the thick coconut milk and simmer on low heat until the curry is thick red golden brown in color. Garnish with chopped coriander leaves.

(When using chili powder, if you like mild flavor, use ½ tsp of chili powder. For medium flavor, uses 1 tsp chili powder, and for hot flavor, use as per the recipe. If you prefer mild curry, use sweet paprika to maintain a bright color and use turmeric for a beautiful golden-orange curry.)

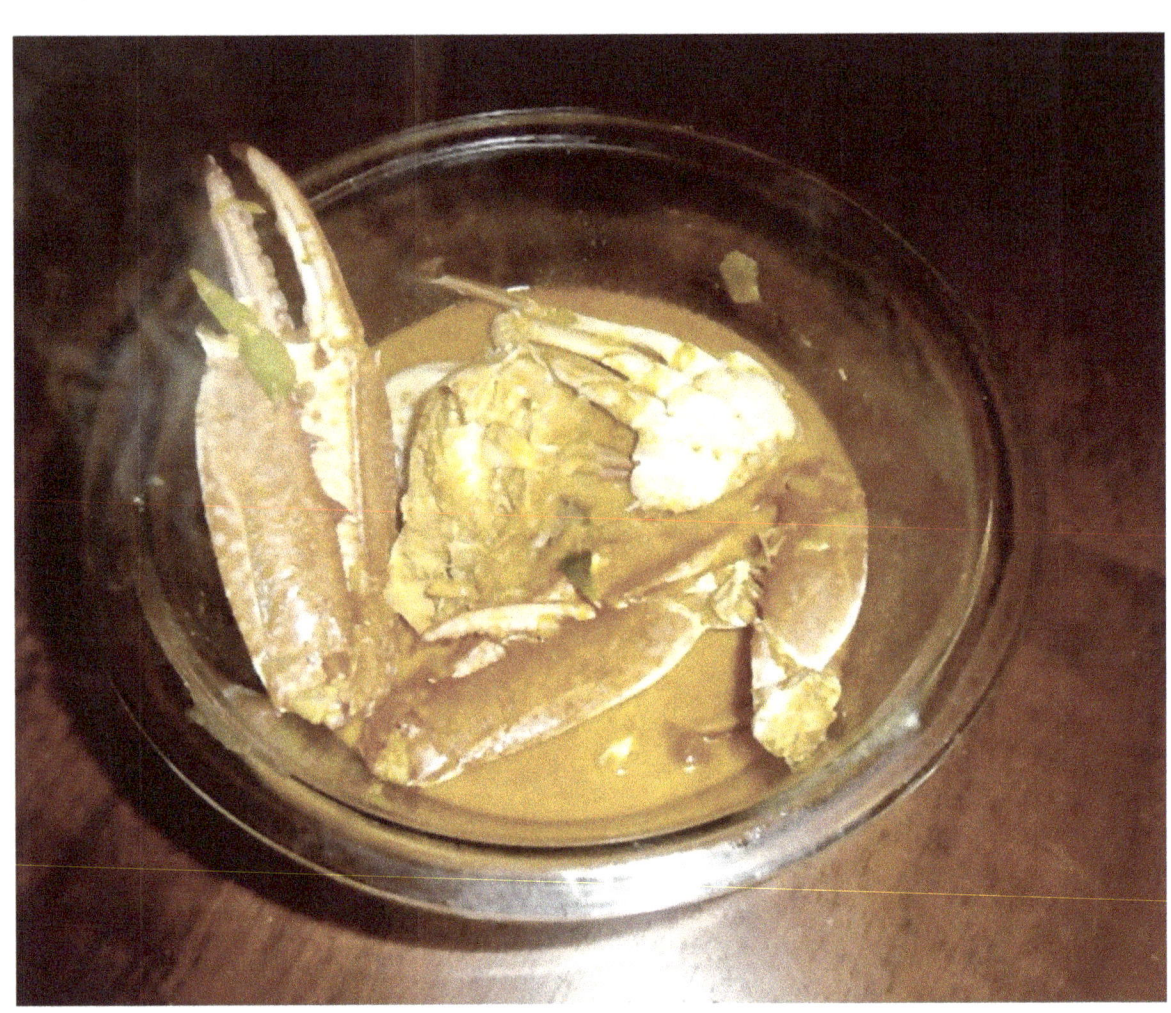

FISH CURRY - (THORA MALU FISH CURRY)

Ingredients:

- 400 Grams Spanish Mackerel Fish (Thora Malu)
- 2 Pieces Goraka –Gamboge
- ½ Onions chopped
- 3 tsp Chili Powder
- 1 tsp Unroasted curry powder
- 1 tsp Pepper powder
- 2 Cloves of Garlic -crushed
- ½ tsp Crushed ginger
- 2 Green chili chopped
- 1 Sprig of Karapincha
- 1 tbs Coconut oil
- 1 1/2 cups Water

Method:

Wash and cut the fish into 1 ½" pieces. Heat coconut oil and add rampe, karapincha, onions, and garlic. Put the fish pieces into a saucepan with all the ingredients and simmer for 20 minutes under low heat. If you like, you can add ½ cup coconut milk to have thick red gravy, or you can leave the curry without adding the coconut milk.

(When using chili powder, if you like mild flavor, use ½ tsp of chili powder. For medium flavor, uses 1 tsp chili powder, and for hot flavor, use as per the recipe. If you prefer mild curry, use sweet paprika to maintain a bright color and use turmeric for a beautiful golden orange curry.)

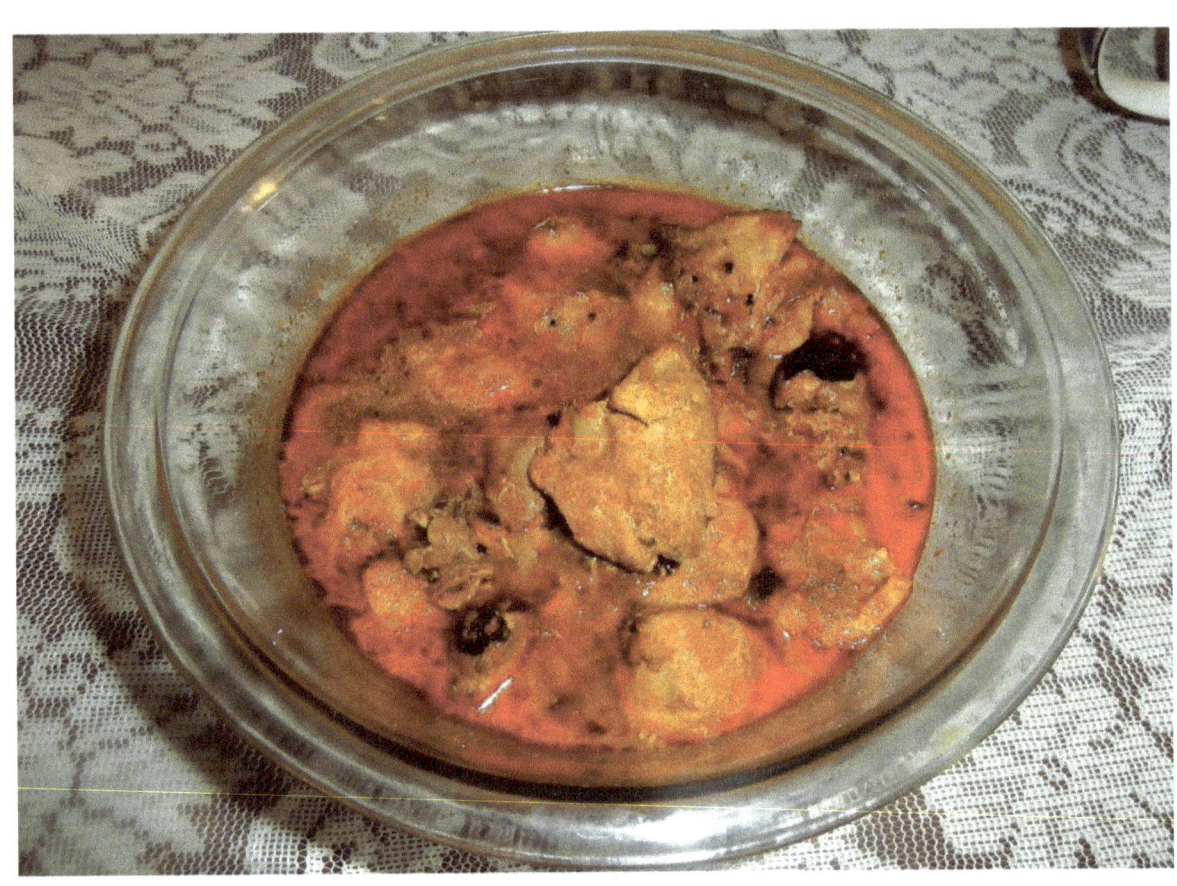

FRIED DRIED FISH

Ingredients:

- 250g Dried fish (Katta dried fish –Katta karawala)
- 1 Large tomato cut into cubes
- 1 Large onion –sliced lengthwise
- 2 Sprig Curry leaves
- 2 Cloves of Garlic- chopped
- 2 Green chilies –chopped
- 2 Capsicums-Malu Miris
- Salt to taste
- 1 tsp Chili powder
- 1 tsp Flaked chili pieces
- 2 tbsp Coconut Oil

Method:

Cut the dried fish into ½" thick pieces. Wash and put the pieces in a saucepan of water just enough to cover the pieces and boil until the pieces are cooked. In a separate frying pan, heat coconut oil and fry onions, chopped green chilies, capsicums , and curry leaves. When onions are browned, add the boiled dried fish, salt, chili powder, and flaked chili pieces. Mix well. Finally add the tomato pieces and let it cook for 2-3 minutes. If the texture of the tempered dry fish is dry, add few more drops of oil to get a rich wet texture.

(When using chili powder, if you like mild flavor, use ½ tsp of chili powder. For medium flavor, use 1 tsp chili powder, and for hot flavor, use as per the recipe. If you prefer mild curry, use sweet paprika to maintain a bright color and use turmeric for a beautiful golden orange curry.)

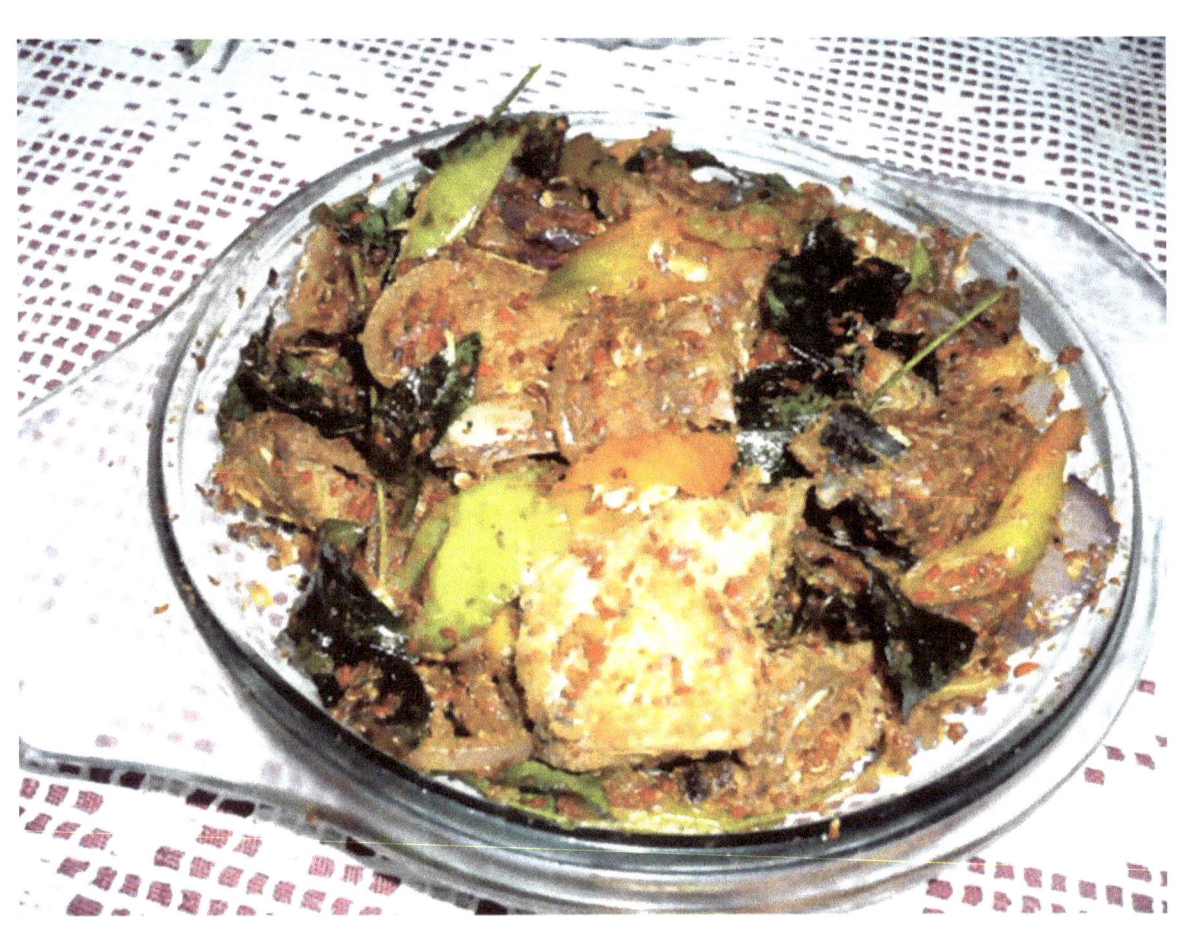

Dinner Ideas

TEMPERED MANIOC OR CASSAVA WITH FISH CURRY

Ingredients:

- 500g Manioc or Cassava
- 2 cloves garlic-chopped
- ¼ Large Onion- chopped
- 1 piece of cinnamon
- 1 Sprig Karapincha Leaves
- 1" piece of rampe
- 1 tsp Mustard seeds
- 3-4 Dried Chillies- broken into large pieces
- Pinch of turmeric
- 2 tbsp. Coconut Oil
- Salt
- ½ Cup scraped Coconut
- Water sufficient to boil jackfruit

Method:

Boil the Manioc or Cassava until it is tender. Drain and add salt and leave it aside. Put 2 tbsp oil in another pan and, once hot, add mustard seeds. When it's popped, add the Karapincha, rampe, onions, cinnamon, garlic, dried chili pieces, and once onions are brown in color, add the boiled jackfruit, saffron, salt, and scraped coconut. Mix well. Allow the coconut to cook for 2-3 minutes.

Serving Ideas:

Meat /Fish curry/Prawns or chicken curry, Lunumiris, Coconut Sambol

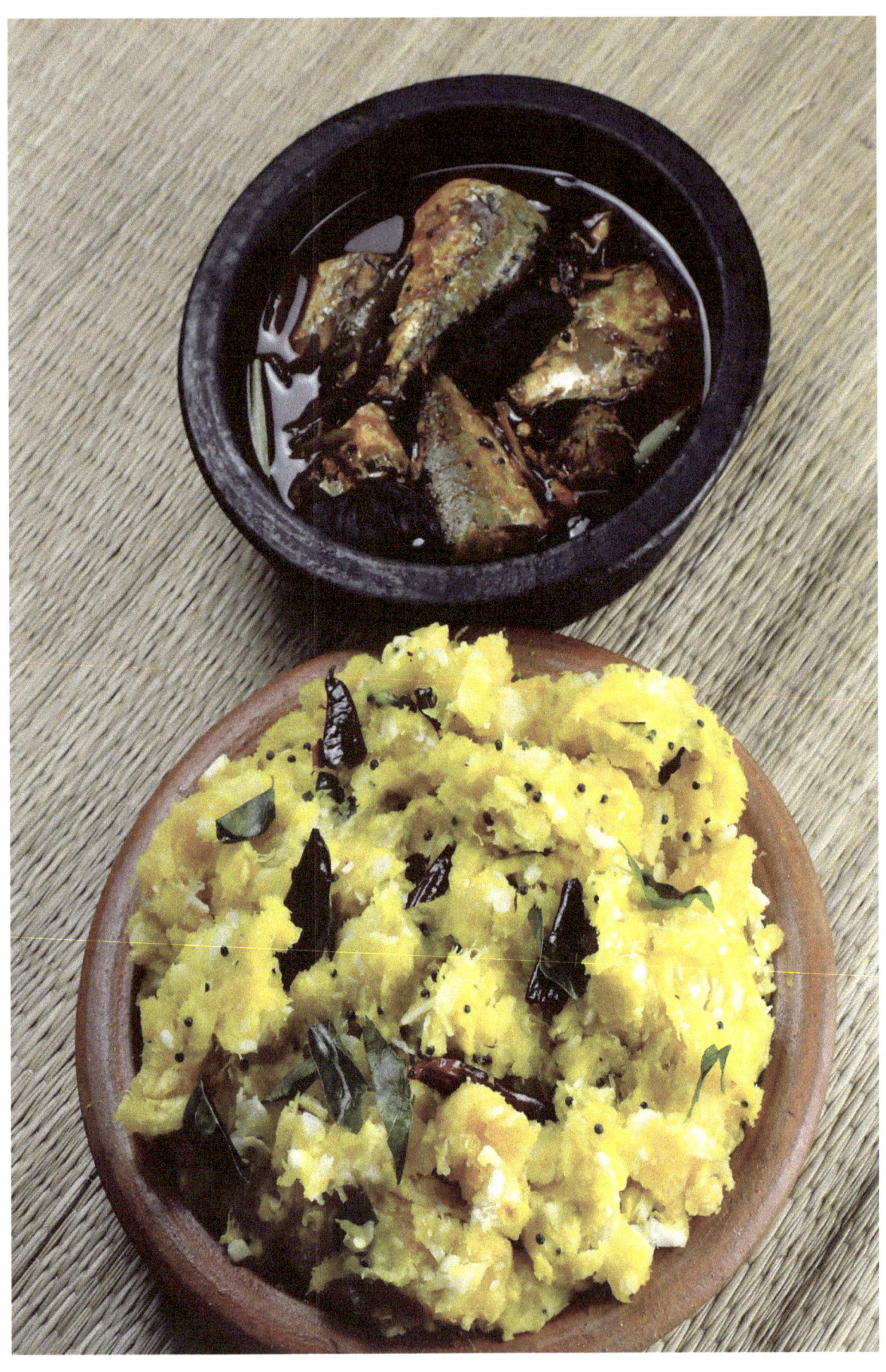

KOTTU ROTI

Roti that is chopped up into little bits and mixed with vegetable, fish, chicken, or eggs is called Kottu Roti.

Ingredients for Chicken Koththu Roti:

- 2 Nos Plain Godhamba Roti- Chopped into small pieces (You can buy plain Godhamba from SriLankan/Indian grocery shops.)
- 1 Medium Onion thinly sliced and halved for decoration.
- 1 Medium Onion- chopped
- ½ tsp Ginger paste
- 1 tsp Garlic paste
- 4 Cloves-Grounded
- 4 Cardamoms-Grounded
- 2 Eggs 100g Leeks
- 100g Carrot
- 1 Sprig Curry leaves
- Salt to taste
- 2 tbsp. Coconut Oil
- 200g Chicken cooked as a curry (See my previous recipe)-Marinated chicken cooked and finalized with coconut milk

Method:

Koththu roti is normally prepared on top of a metal board, and the ingredients are chopped using 2 metal pieces. You can use a BBQ cooking top or use a flat cooking pan for cooking. Chop the Godhamba roti into small pieces. Prepare a chicken curry, as I have mentioned in my previous recipes. (Marinated chicken cooked and finalized by coconut milk.). Heat some coconut oil and saute garlic, ginger, curry leaves, and add two eggs. Cook for a while. Then add onions, leeks, and carrots. Mix them well. Sri Lankans normally beat the metal boards hard on the ingredients to mix and chop the ingredients finely. If you don't have this opportunity, chop the ingredients finely and mix well. Blend all ingredients together and allow them to cook for 2- 3 minutes. Repeat the process of mixing (chopping) until the vegetables are slightly cooked. Then add the chopped roti, mix well. Finalize with the chicken curry. Chop the chicken into small chunks and remove bones. Add ½ cup chicken gravy and chicken pieces into the mixture and blend well. Serve as a pyramid, towering with Sri Lankan flavors, such as onion ring halves, Leek strands, karapincha, etc. You will love this.

If you like Fish koththu, you can add a fish curry with small broken fish pieces instead of chicken curry. Prepare the fish curry as per the given recipe for Fish Curry.

If you like Egg Koththu, add 2 beaten eggs instead of chicken curry and let it cook for 2-3 minutes before mixing.

If you like vegetable kottu, don't add any meat or fish and serve as it is.

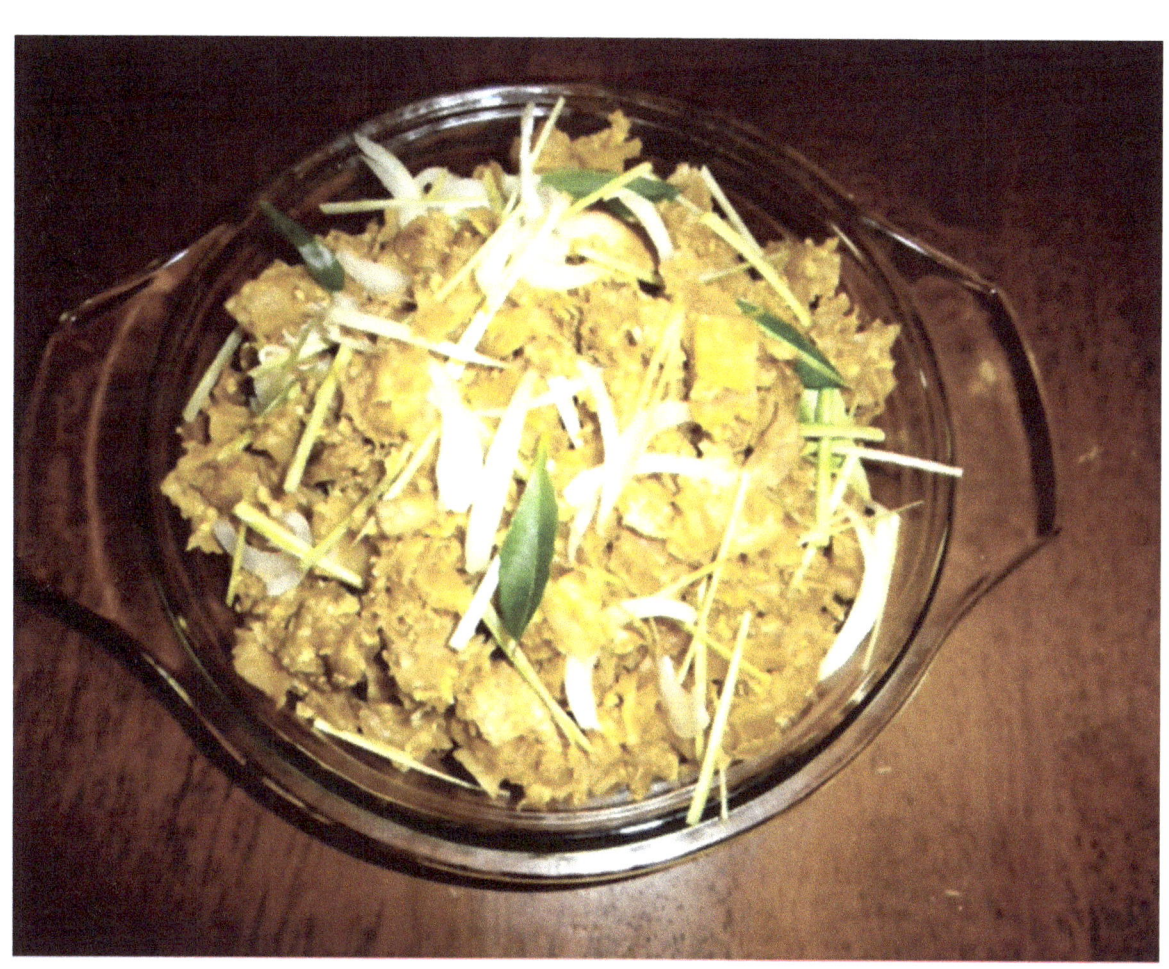

Desserts

WATALAPPUM

Ingredients:

- 250g Jaggery
- 5 Eggs
- 2 ½ cups Thick Coconut Milk
- 25g Cashew Nuts
- Few Drops of Vanilla Essence
- 1/2 tsp Mixed Spices

Method:

Put the jaggery and coconut milk in a pan and heat it under low heat until jaggery is dissolved in coconut milk. Beat eggs well until it doesn't fall when turned upside down. Add milk and jaggery mixture little by little to the egg mixture and continue beating. Add powdered spices and vanilla and beat well. Pour into ceramic/ glass bowl and decorate with cashew nut halves. Cover top with oil paper or aluminum foil and steam or bake at 170-190c (350-375 f) for 45 to 50 minutes.

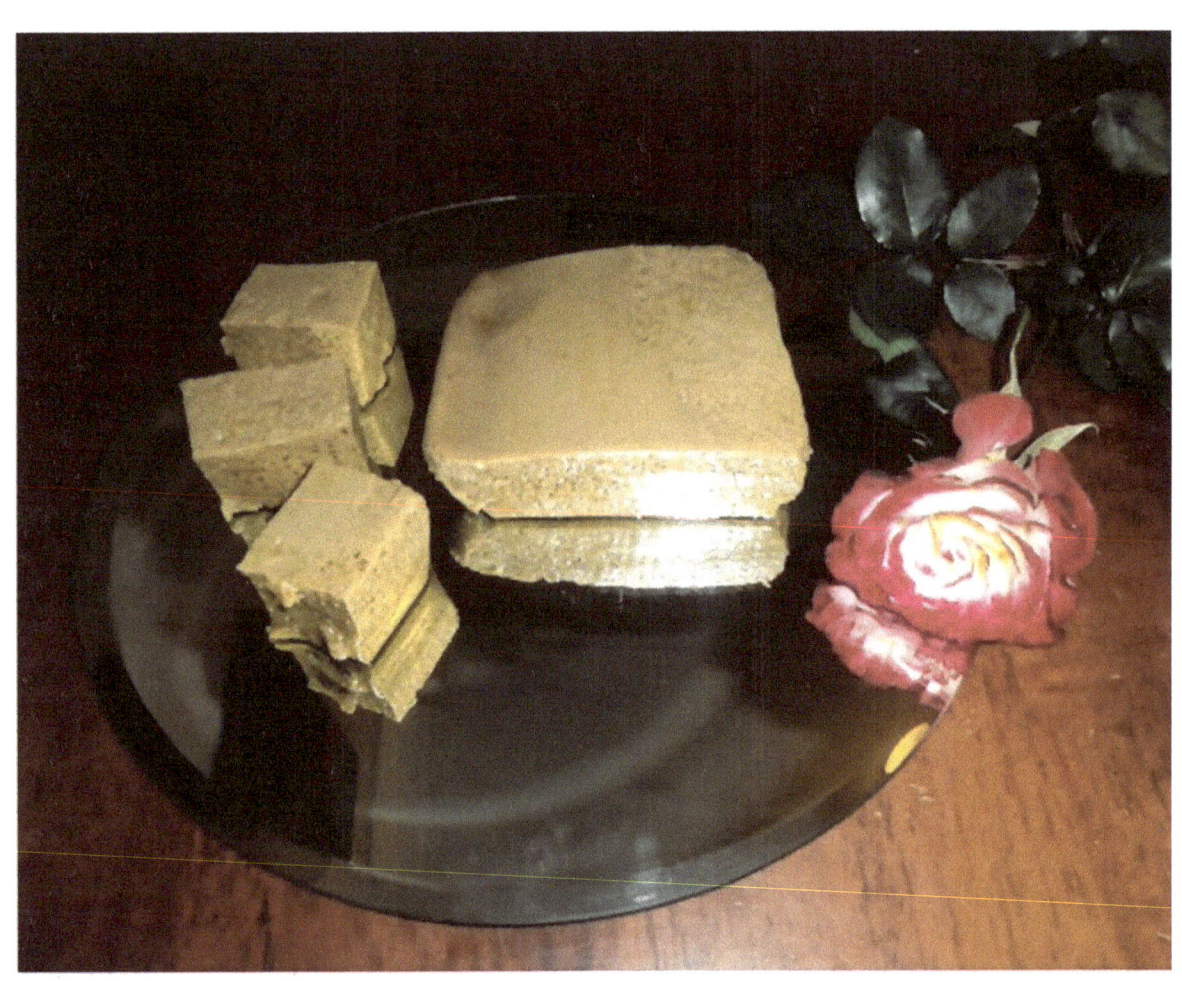

CHOCOLATE MARIE BISCUIT PUDDING

Ingredients:

- 250 g Butter
- 320 g Caster Sugar
- 2 Eggs
- 100g Cocoa Powder
- 1 Tsp Vanilla Essence
- 50g Chopped Baked Cashew Nuts
- 200g Marie Biscuits
- 1 Cup of milk to dip the Marie Biscuits.

Method:

Beat butter and sugar until sugar is dissolved.

Add 2 eggs and beat until they are creamy.

Add the 100g Cocoa Powder and Vanilla Essence and beat.

Add one layer of chocolate mixture into a Pyrex bowl.

Dip the Marie Biscuits in milk and spread one layer on top of the chocolate mixture.

Repeat Chocolate mixture and Marie biscuits layering.

Repeat the process until the chocolate mixture is over. (Include at least 4 layers of Marie Biscuits).

On top of the final layer, add crumbled Marie Biscuits and chopped roasted cashew nuts. Refrigerate to set the pudding for 2 hours.

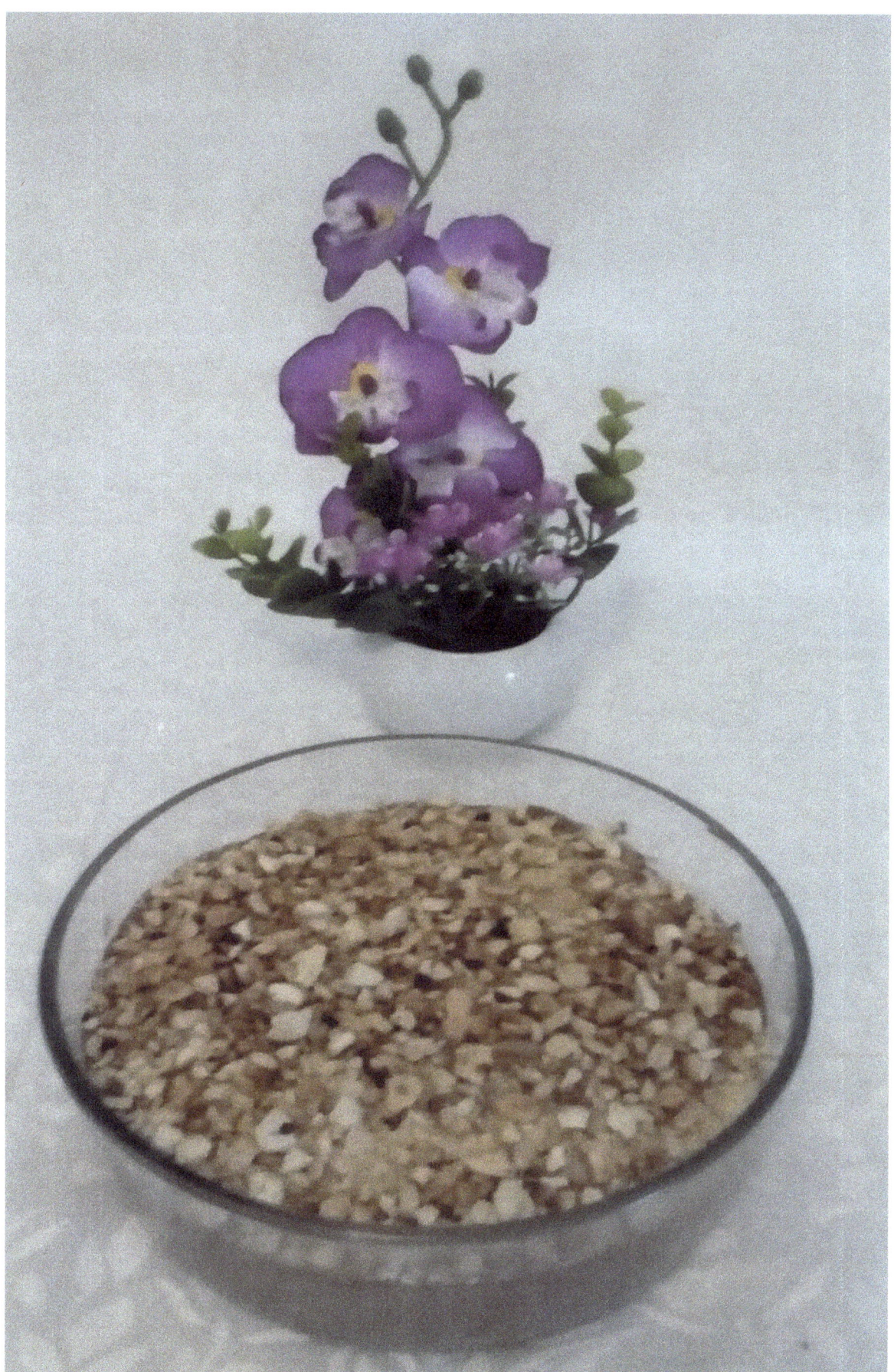

www.ingramcontent.com/pod-product-compliance
Lightning Source LLC
Chambersburg PA
CBHW061757290426
44109CB00030B/2882